skilful

skilful living

integrated health for busy people

Carl Lyons

MIDDLESEX
UNIVERSITY
PRESS

First published in 2004 by Middlesex University Press

ISBN 1 904750 08 7

A CIP catalogue record for this book is available from
The British Library

Cover design by Bluemove Communications

Book design by Helen Taylor

Printed in the UK by The Alden Group, Oxford

Middlesex University Press, Queensway, Enfield, Middlesex EN4 3SF

Tel: +44 (0)20 8411 5734: +44 (0)20 8880 4262 Fax: +44 (0)20 8411 5736

www.mupress.co.uk

This book is dedicated to

Jordana, my daughter and constant inspiration

Acknowledgements

A warm thank you to my friend and fellow adventurer, Marcus Walia, who developed the yoga routine and illustrated the desktop yoga. Also to Peter Critten for his inspiration and support throughout the writing of this book. Thanks also to Celia Cozens for her clear and honest editing and for challenging me to be more skilful.

contents

introduction

OUR HEALTH IS THE SPRINGBOARD for everything we do in life. By optimising our health it is possible to achieve extraordinary things in every other area of our lives, consistently, measurably and permanently. Most of us want to change, to live our lives expressing our full potential, but many don't know how. This book is about providing practical tools and techniques to identify the things you want to achieve and make them a reality in your life. Whether the things you desire are professional or personal, big or small does not matter. For any change we need energy, focus and desire and this is where health becomes important. By achieving your own optimum levels of health you will feel you can achieve just about anything.

This material takes a fundamental look at all the factors that influence your health and integrates them into a system that supports your natural cycles, gives you consistently high levels of performance and allows you to live life with spectacular levels of energy, health and vitality. I believe this is how we are meant to live – without constraint or limitation. I describe here a system that can change your life for the better – if you choose to apply the principles. I know this to be true because it has transformed my life, and the lives of many other people. Through personal and group consultations many people have created changes that are life enhancing and permanent.

The uniqueness of the system lies in its comprehensive approach to health; it examines diet and nutrition, exercise habits, natural life cycles and mental and emotional processes. It draws knowledge and wisdom from traditional health systems including Ayurveda and yoga as well as more conventional practices and takes the best and most practical aspects of each system to produce a totally integrated lifestyle approach called Skilful Living.

Skilful Living is summarised under three pillars: Skilful Eating, Skilful

Activity and Skilful Thinking. Individually each pillar will provide practical tools that provide measurable benefits. However, the true power lies in an integration of the three, providing you with a complete system for simultaneously improving health and performance in every important area of your life.

The system is called Skilful Living because it requires aware and deliberate application.

When we do anything with skill, whether in sport, business or simply everyday life, then we consistently do a number of things:

● Get very clear about the desired outcome and understand and discriminate efficiently between the options presented. Skilful people process and act on this information quickly.

● Control our responses effectively. This may be a physical or mental ability that is applied directly to provide us with outcomes we desire, such as hitting a golf ball or focusing our thoughts.

● Take consistent action. Skilful people do things over and over until the first two steps become unconscious.

By applying these steps to a definite goal the outcomes become more predictable.

Nothing in this material is described as right or wrong but as 'skilful' or 'unskilful' in as much as it is related to your desired outcomes. Eating, activity or thinking are considered as being skilful if they take you a step closer to achieving your goal or vision, to becoming that person you wish to be. Unskilful behaviour is that which is inconsistent with your personal vision.

The book is therefore divided into the following three sections:

Under **Skilful Eating** we will examine:

● How food influences energy levels and performance
● Understanding your personal food history
● Assessing your digestion
● Learning to listen to your body
● The when and how of eating
● Balanced nutrition and food for constitutions

Under **Skilful Activity** we will examine:

● Aligning your activities with nature's cycles for activity, eating and sleeping

- Ayurvedic daily routines
- The power of exercise – fitting a short and simple yoga routine into your life
- The power of breath – breathing exercises for managing stress and anxiety
- Desktop yoga – prevention and treatment of common work-related complaints
- Understanding your mind/body type and how it influences your life and work

Under **Skilful Thinking** we will examine:

- How your thoughts create your experiences
- Getting clear about what you want to be, do and have
- Fitness advice for the mind – increasing awareness and concentration
- Creating a vision for your life and making it happen
- Practical goal setting and visualisation

The Skilful Eating and Skilful Activity sections of this system are about providing you with the optimum level of physical resource to live to your full potential. Skilful Thinking provides you with the mental and creative resources to construct a life of your own design. Consider your body as the vehicle that houses this creation equipment. Without your physical and mental energies working at their optimum and in an integrated way, you will not meet your true potential. True health is about our mental, emotional and spiritual selves; it is about growth, purpose and contribution. Once we have true consistency between these elements of our lives, then we can live with breathtaking clarity.

This is about integrating your life at every level and needs a degree of mental and emotional awareness that is available to everybody, but mastered by few. You will need to decide whether you are prepared to do whatever it takes to attain this level of control over your life. If you are, then I guarantee the rewards will be worth it.

Using this book

This book is designed to be a practical workbook. It is punctuated with exercises for you to complete before you move onto the next section.

The exercises are all indicated by a text box

Try and build the exercises into your current daily routine. You will find that it is possible to make small changes that create a big difference to your energy and outlook. It is designed to be integrated into your current life and help you make an even greater contribution to what you are already doing. Our modern lifestyle means that we are all busy people, but at the same time our expectations of the things we wish to experience have become much greater. These two things, less time and greater personal desires, do not need to be mutually exclusive. By using our resources a little more skilfully, we can design and achieve the lifestyle we truly deserve.

Skilful Living is about setting clear life goals and then developing a strategy to achieve them by consciously applying the tools and techniques to make that vision real. We will examine our physical health, but we will also look at some of our fundamental thinking and feeling processes, asking why we think the way we do and more importantly whether thinking and behaving in this way serves us in a positive and purposeful way.

The approach we will take is simple. You will analyse where you are now in terms of your health, create a vision of where you want to be and then bridge any gap with some practical tools and techniques. Be open-minded, experimental and curious; challenge yourself to think about approaching your life in a different way.

Integrated health

In our society we often take a very fragmented approach to life. We compartmentalise our responsibilities, often stretching our personal resources to the limit, creating imbalance and ultimately illness. As far as our health is concerned we cannot fragment our lives. If we are under pressure at work it spills over into our personal life, and vice versa. This often becomes an unhealthy, self-supporting cycle. The work ethic, particularly in certain western countries, means that we work long hard hours and are regularly under pressure. Because of this we often skip lunch or take it on the go, drinking plenty of coffee or tea to keep our energy levels high. Many of us work late and have difficulty leaving the pressures of the day behind. This affects our personal relationships and the energy we have available to devote to them. Often after a poor night's sleep because of the pressure, anxiety and our eating habits we start the cycle all over again. Under these circumstances we easily lose sight of the bigger picture and feel that work totally dominates our life, our choices and our sense of freedom.

We will look at replacing this cycle with something that is a lot more supportive of our health and actively makes use of our natural functional and energetic cycles. Our health has a direct impact on each of the different roles we have in life and for that reason we need to take a much more holistic approach, while at the same time practically and sensibly integrating the principles with these other responsibilities. It is not necessary to turn life upside-down: the lifestyle adjustments described need not be dramatic, but they may be life changing.

Integrated health is the balanced use of all of our personal resources as well as the practical application of tools and techniques from a number of different health systems. It takes the best and most practical elements from each and through practical experience combines them in a powerful and accessible way.

Ayurveda is the oldest and most complete health system in the world and is an important cornerstone of this programme. As well as using the wisdom of Ayurveda, Skilful Living has blended it with practices such as yoga, relaxation and visualisation as well as diet and nutrition. In the next section I will explain in greater detail about Ayurveda, how it fits with our modern lifestyle and how we have made a powerful system even stronger with the integration of these other practices. The power of Ayurveda lies in its practical application and the fact that it works. We will determine your personal constitution, or mind/body type and use this information to manage your health, energy and relationships, both in your personal and professional life.

Why bother at all?

How many of us are living a life entirely of our own design? Almost every single person I have met in my training seminars and personal consultations desires improvement in some area of their lives. Those living their life successfully have a sense of purpose and contribution in life that flows from their basic nature. They feel in control of their life experiences and are invariably excited about the possibilities that these experiences bring. I have found that what most people ultimately consider as success is a sense of personal fulfilment, health, quality of relationships and life direction. The more material factors either matter less or naturally flow from this state.

There seem to be two significant factors that contribute to our level of happiness in life: one of these is measured by how much in control of our lives we feel, and the other is the degree to which we are growing in life. The first of these is not about control in a constraining, constricting way, it is about how well we manage the cause-and-effect relationships that give us our life experiences; the feeling of being in creative control of our own destiny. The second, growth, and ultimately contribution, is also a fundamental necessity for us as human beings. No matter how much 'stuff' we may have, if we are not expanding our consciousness in some way, then unhappiness is the result.

I changed my own life experiences by learning and understanding what others have already done and by finding what really works. This modelling process does not give you exactly what others have, it allows you to develop the level of consciousness experienced by them, providing you with your own unique version of those experiences.

Some years ago, I felt like I was living somebody else's life. It was not that my work or relationships were disastrous, rather that they weren't the best they could be. I knew that life could be so much more but was not sure how to bring about the changes. There was no life-threatening condition that would spur me into activity, no spectre of poverty or starvation. I'd never been a complete failure, I'd done better than some, and worse than others. Should I not be content with what I had gained, or should I risk what I had achieved for a vague and uncertain 'more'? I just did not know, and the weight of the dilemma anchored me firmly in immobility and indecision.

I knew, however, that if I didn't change I was destined to continue living a life of compromise, never achieving the things of which I knew I was capable. It was then that I made a decision. A decision that I was going to actively take control of my life and not compromise on achieving my goals. I searched my life experiences to discover what I was really passionate about, then followed my discoveries through with action. I left my job and went to study Ayurveda and yoga in India and the UK.

I became clearer about who I was and where I was going. Although I did have a profound moment of insight, none of these changes occurred in a flash of enlightenment. The lasting changes took tenacity, belief and commitment. I believe we have to make things happen by living a life that integrates our thoughts, words and actions to actively create the life we want. Such magnificent aspirations are not exclusively for the great and the famous, everybody has the faculty to make such choices and changes in their lives. It is our very purpose. Skilful Living is a result of my personal process. I describe it here in the hope that you will cast off the limitations of your conditioning and live to your full potential.

The benefits I have gained are to do with my personal fulfilment, health, quality of relationships and life direction. I am now doing what I love to do in life, the people around me inspire and energise me and I am moving always closer to living my own personal dream. I have rediscovered my passion and purpose in life and am actively living it.

This passion is to help others realise their full potential and make lasting and measurable differences in their lives. If you are ready to start designing the life you want and are prepared to undergo the changes necessary, then this book has arrived with you at just the right moment. It does not matter whether the desired change is to be a better employee, parent, sportsperson or life partner, Skilful Living, applied with commitment, can make a difference.

The three pillars of skilful living

i Skilful eating

Our eating habits are so fundamental to improving our personal achievement and performance that they are often overlooked. The digestion of food takes more energy than anything else you do; more than swimming, cycling, running or any other exercise. Energy is a little like money, no matter how much you have you can always use a little more. By understanding how your body responds to the food you put in it and by working with your natural needs you can achieve spectacular energy levels and states of health. When Ayurveda deals with food, it discusses not only what to eat, but also when, how and where. Under what is called the 'eightfold discipline of food' it discusses all these elements, helping to define an eating plan that is right for each individual. We will talk about lifestyle plans, not short-term changes. In this section we won't be discussing temporary fixes or diets, we will be addressing your fundamental relationship with food; why you eat the way you do and how to change it forever. This will involve reconnecting with your own body, getting in touch with your senses and using the natural messages that are constantly being transmitted; then using these messages to respond actively, thereby designing your levels of energy, concentration and focus.

ii Skilful activity

This relates to our behaviour in life. It includes physical exercise and how our bodies are designed for movement. We will identify the natural energy cycles described by Ayurveda so that you can actively utilise them, making them work for you rather than against you. We will provide a simple but powerful yoga routine that is guaranteed to make a big difference to your level of health. It is a 15-minute sequence consisting of postures, breathing and relaxation and is suitable for everyone, regardless of experience or physical fitness. Under Skilful Activity we will also examine your working life and how it affects your health. We will learn how certain foods, emotions, relationships and work circumstances affect your well-being – how they can ultimately manifest as disease – and what to do about it. We will also look at constitutions in the workplace. How certain mind/body types have particular strengths and inclinations and how to use this information for actively managing relationships at work.

iii Skilful thinking

The first two pillars provide you with the physical and energetic resources to apply the third. The way that we organise our thinking processes drives everything else we do, including our eating and activities. We will discuss how we have developed our current thinking habits through our conditioning processes and you will have an opportunity to decide whether these habits serve you. Do they deliver the life you desire? We will look at some practical tools for breaking through this conditioning, associating with more positive behaviours. By aligning your thoughts with your values and vision, miraculous things can occur in your life. We will set goals and then use visualisation to focus your thoughts and your vision, thus harnessing your more subtle intuitive forces as well as your intellectual resources.

Inspiring permanent change

Everything outlined in this book is about making permanent change. We are often encouraged to adopt a survival mentality in our behaviour, concentrating on the short term at the expense of the long term.

The other approach that we will take is to concentrate on the positive, not manage the negative. This is not a therapy book, it is about managing health, not tackling illness.

For making these fundamental changes we will adopt a model that is simple but effective:

Step 1 - Understand who and where you are now

You will undertake exercises that will assess your health, identify your values and beliefs, and establish your personal constitution. These are all pieces of the same jigsaw puzzle to build a detailed picture of your current physical and mental make-up.

Step 2 - Develop a vision of the future

Success in anything we do is directly related to clarity of purpose. It is essential to develop a crystal-clear vision of the future if you are to make it a reality. Towards the end of the book I provide some exercises to help you develop this clarity of vision. Most of us have dreams and aspirations when we are children that get lost through the frustration of our daily existence. Living skilfully is about living consciously and imaginatively. Consciousness and imagination are powerful tools that many of us lose the sense of how to use effectively as we grow older.

Consider managing your life the way you would manage other important projects. This requires three things: a clear understanding of your starting point, a vision of the future and a strategy to take you there.

Step 3 - Apply the strategy

If there is a performance gap between steps 1 and 2, then the tension that is created is called desire to change. The three pillars are the tools that, when applied to your life, provide a strategy for bridging this gap.

Having generated the desire for change, it is important that we apply the tools to take the first steps and also maintain momentum. I will be describing proven methods that can make big differences, even in some cases with small adjustments to your routine, eating habits, thinking or behaviour. We are characterised by the things that we do consistently in life, not by those that we do every now and again. So we need to apply the tools and techniques in an integrated, consistent way to get the most benefit.

The final step in this whole model is that of action. The ultimate result of our work will be a new behaviour, driven perhaps by new thinking or beliefs and new knowledge. But we must ultimately act.

Raise your standards

We are often challenged in our society to accept much less than we are capable of. This is particularly true where our health is concerned. The emphasis in our culture is on disease rather than health. If you think about it, we have a National Disease Service rather than a National Health Service. This is not a criticism, it is a simple observation. This emphasis on the cure of illness rather than the promotion of health leads us to concentrate on the negative, rather than the positive. If you go to your GP, feeling somewhat under the weather; perhaps your energy is low, your digestion not so good, your sleep and concentration is poor and you catch more than your fair share of colds – he or she will undertake a series of tests. Often the tests will yield nothing and in the absence of any discernible disease your doctor will declare you to be healthy. But health is not the absence of disease. You know you are not healthy, but the messages you are given from those around you are that it could be much worse, or there is always someone else worse off. So our social conditioning lowers our expectations of our performance.

We should demand the best level of health that we are capable of as individuals, all of the time, without compromise.

This is our right and it is the standard that our bodies were designed to achieve. This goes not only for our health, but every other area of our life performance. A number of years ago I did not feel in control of my life, I felt like I was being carried along by forces that were seemingly out of my control. The most significant thing that I did to help change my circumstances and take control was to raise my standards. This was a choice. A decision I made in the moment. I listed the things that I would not tolerate any more and those I wanted in my life. Then I refused to compromise in achieving these goals. This simple step can be instantly life changing; but nothing will happen unless you believe that it's possible.

Believe you can do it

You can make lists of things until you run out of paper, but if you don't have belief in yourself to achieve your goals, nothing will happen. We somehow need to get ourselves to the point where we believe with every fibre of our being that we are capable of great achievements and that they will definitely occur. This means taking a fundamental look at our values and deep thought processes.

Our values shape who we are, how we behave and what we achieve. We will examine your values and beliefs in more detail later, but it is worth reminding ourselves that for many of us, our most fundamental belief processes are formed at an early stage in our lives, often through a process of conditioning. This means that much of our thinking is influenced by others and we rarely revisit them to ask if these beliefs still serve us. If you have ever found yourself in a situation where you have difficulty deciding something, it is because you are not clear about what you value most. The process we will undertake in Skilful Thinking is to get very clear about our current values and whether they provide us with the experiences we desire in our life. We will link these with our vision of the future and attempt to make powerful, positive associations with their achievement. This gives us some strong reasons why we want to achieve our goals. Up to now you may not have acted simply because you did not have a strong enough reason to.

Design your change to be consistent with your own goals rather than leaving it to circumstances, or worse in the hands of others who have a vested interest in how you think.

I've met many people who have made significant changes in their lives as a result of traumatic experiences. In these cases, change is usually painful and driven by an external, unplanned event. Very often the changes have ultimately produced life-enhancing results, which proved to those involved they were capable of things they otherwise would not have believed. However, when we live skilfully, we don't wait for the traumatic event! Decide to take control of your life now.

How healthy are you?

The following questionnaire is not designed as a comprehensive health check, but as a guide to concentrate your energy in the areas of most benefit. Answer each question by placing a number in each box:

0 = Never/Rarely

1 = Sometimes

2 = Always/Frequently

eating

1   Do you suffer from bloating or excess belching?

2   Do you suffer from pain or heartburn after eating?

3   Do you suffer from diarrhoea or constipation?

4   Are your bowel movements irregular? (less than once per day)

5   Do you have bad breath or a bitter taste in your mouth?

6   Do you eat until you feel full?

7   Do you eat less than 5 portions of fresh fruit or veg each day?

8   Do you drink less than 1.5 litres of water each day?

9   Do you drink coffee or alcohol daily?

10 Do you have difficulty digesting certain foods?

Total for Eating

activity

1   Are you physically inactive? (less than 3 times per week)

2   Are you sluggish on waking?

3   Does your work leave you feeling stressed and drained?

4   How often do you find yourself yawning through the day?

5   Do you have energy dips after eating?

6   Do you find you need frequent chocolate or sugar breaks?

7   Do you have less energy than you need for your activities?

8   Do you have difficulty sleeping?

9   Is your daily cycle exhausting?

10 Do you eat late in the evening or at night? (after about 8 o'clock)

Total for Activity

thinking

1   Do you get confused or find it hard to concentrate?

2   Has your memory deteriorated or is your short-term memory poor?

3   Do you have a feeling of depression or hopelessness?

4   Do you get anxious easily, have panic attacks or over-react to stress?

5   Do you suffer from mood swings or get angry or irritable?

6   Is your sleep disturbed due to anxiety?

7   Do you have difficulty relaxing or leaving work behind?

8   Do you feel you have lost your direction in life?

9   Do you suffer from low self-esteem?

10 Do you put other people first in your relationships?

Total for Thinking

general immunity

1   Do you smoke?

2   Do you suffer from headaches or migraines?

3   Do you have watery, itchy eyes?

4   Do you have sinus problems, ear infections or itchy ears?

5   Do you have skin problems like acne, flaky skin or rashes?

6   Do you suffer from excess sweat or body odour?

7   Do you have aches or pains in your joints or muscles?

8   Do you suffer from more than 3 colds a year?

9   Are you prone to or have difficulty shifting infections?

10 Do you often need to take drugs or medicines?

Total for General Immunity

Total for all sections

If you scored 8 or more in any one section, you probably need to concentrate your efforts on that pillar. A score of 35 or more in total, or a high score in the general immunity check means that you are better undertaking the whole programme and making changes in all three pillars. This exercise should give you an idea of where to focus your efforts. If there is a difference between your current levels of health and your ideal levels then this is good news. This difference should generate an important emotion within you: desire. If we have a strong enough reason, we can achieve anything.

If you choose, make this the start of a journey of self-discovery. Before you embark on the journey, I want you to answer these questions:

What area of my life would I most like to improve?

...and why?

Your Ayurvedic constitution

According to Ayurvedic philosophy we are all born with a constitutional type, which is established at the moment of our conception and stays with us until death. This natural disposition, although fixed throughout life, is often masked by more superficial changes, which often result in imbalance or illness. By understanding our most fundamental nature, we are able to adjust our behaviour and work in harmony with our physical and mental needs. So, understanding our constitution in some detail helps us to identify our natural tendencies, our body type, how we respond to certain stimuli and our thinking style. Skilfully used, this information can help to transform our performance. In a moment we will assess your constitution, but first we need to learn some more about the system upon which it is based.

Ayurveda – the science of living

'Ayurveda' is a Sanskrit word derived from two roots: 'ayus' meaning *life* and 'vid' meaning *knowledge* or *science*. Therefore, the word Ayurveda means the *knowledge* or the *science of life*.

It is a fitting meaning for a very complete system, the oldest complete health system in the world dating back more than 3,000 years. Ayurveda was conceived as an ancient Indian healing tradition to support individuals in pursuit of their personal goals in life: earning a living, contributing to society and supporting a family. Fundamental to this aim was the knowledge that none of this is possible without good health throughout life. This is a very practical outlook. It recognises that we do have responsibilities in life that have to be fulfilled, and that health and longevity are the foundations upon which these aims are achieved.

Ayurveda is primarily a system of health promotion, but also has a detailed scientific methodology for the treatment of disease. This emphasis on prevention means that a very proactive approach is taken towards maintaining all aspects of health: physical, emotional and mental. It tells us which substances, qualities and actions are life-enhancing and which are not. It provides detailed advice on daily and seasonal lifestyle factors such as diet, exercise and general activities including oral hygiene, self-massage and many others. It has a huge array of herbal medicines used in the cure of disease and rejuvenation treatments. It is responsible for an increasingly popular form of purification therapy called Panchakarma and was the first system to develop inoculations and practise plastic surgery.

Its effectiveness has been proven in India over thousands of years on millions of people and it is now becoming very popular in the west due to its practical application and extremely powerful results. Its focus is very clearly on the health and longevity of the individual and it is for these reasons we have used its principles as one of the corner stones of Skilful Living. Ayurveda is a very deep and complex science and this book is in no way meant to provide the reader with a comprehensive understanding. I have taken here some of the most practical elements of the preventative side of Ayurveda that in my experience provide definite results. We don't discuss the underlying philosophy here or the vast therapeutic side of the science.

Swasthavrittam is a Sanskrit word that refers to activities that support health and includes: *ahara* (food), *vihara* (activity) and *vichaara* (thinking).

This forms the basis for our three pillars, which are made even more effective when combined with the other practices I describe. It is the application of these that will form the strategy for your change.

The three doshas

Fundamental to the philosophy of Ayurveda is the existence of three energy forces or doshas. These are called *vata*, *pitta* and *kapha*. Health exists when all three doshas are in balance and conversely all disease is a result of imbalance. The doshas exist at a physical, functional and mental level in our bodies. Each dosha has particular qualities and responsibilities in the body and also specific manifestations in a balanced and imbalanced state. These are the qualities and functions of the three doshas:

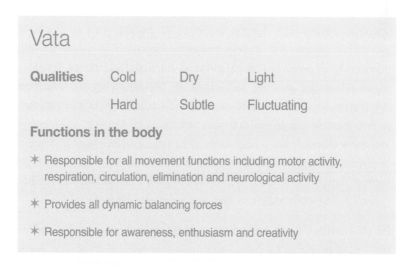

Vata

Qualities	Cold	Dry	Light
	Hard	Subtle	Fluctuating

Functions in the body

* Responsible for all movement functions including motor activity, respiration, circulation, elimination and neurological activity

* Provides all dynamic balancing forces

* Responsible for awareness, enthusiasm and creativity

Pitta

Qualities	Moist	Intense	Sharp	Hot
	Light	Odorous	Liquid	

Functions in the body

* Responsible for all transformations including digestion, metabolism and intelligence

* Driving force for assertiveness, intensity and responsible for sense of vision

* Promotes bodily heat, lustre and complexion

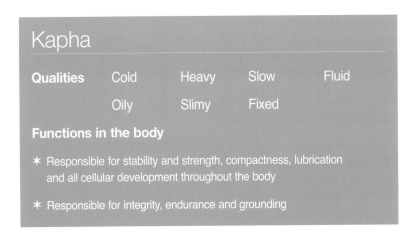

Kapha

Qualities   Cold   Heavy   Slow   Fluid

                Oily   Slimy   Fixed

Functions in the body

✳ Responsible for stability and strength, compactness, lubrication
  and all cellular development throughout the body

✳ Responsible for integrity, endurance and grounding

The three doshas are entirely interdependent and together govern all of the
activities of life. Understanding the individual qualities is important and the
above descriptions will become clearer as we make some practical
applications later on.

Determining your Ayurvedic constitution

The three doshas exist throughout the body and combine uniquely at
conception to create our personal constitution. Our Ayurvedic constitution
relates to our basic nature and reflects our preferences and tendencies at a
physical, functional and mental level. So, Ayurveda views each person as
individual but uses broad categories based upon dominant dosha or a
combination of the doshas and it is this characterisation that we call
constitution, or your mind/body type.

Seven combinations are considered:

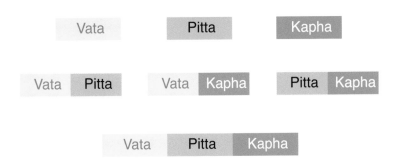

Knowing your constitution will allow you to predict your response to
certain potentially stressful situations both in general and particularly in the

workplace. With a little practice, you will also be able to characterise those around you: colleagues, customers and family. This may be helpful in understanding your relationship with them a little better by being aware of the things that motivate them from a basic needs level. However, constitution does not explain everything about a person, it describes preferences we have and if used well it can help us to improve our own lives and the lives of others around us.

Let us now determine your own personal constitution by completing the following questionnaire. Tick the description that best fits a description of you. Don't take too long in deciding each one, try to be as spontaneous as you can. If you really cannot decide on one description think back to your most natural inclination, perhaps when you were a child, or how you have reacted in general throughout your lifetime. Where categories have fluctuated greatly then choose the right-hand column even if it does not accurately describe you now. In some cases, if more than one description fits, tick them both. Avoid the temptation to mark yourself as you would like to be rather than as you are. Consider getting somebody else to complete the questionnaire for you and then compare the two to give greater clarity. Add up the ticks in each column until you have three numbers at the end of the table.

Determining Your Mind/Body Type ▶

Physical

Body frame	Large boned, easily puts on weight	Medium with good muscle	Small with difficulty putting on weight
Height	Short and sturdy or tall and sturdy	Medium	Very short or very tall
Joints	Big, well formed and lubricated	Normal, well proportioned	Prominent and dry
Muscular structure	Large and thick	Medium, well formed and firm	Prominent tendons
Skin texture	Thick, oily, cold	Soft, lustrous, warm with moles or freckles	Dry, cool
Veins	Not visible	Evenly distributed	Easily visible
Hair	Thick, lustrous, plentiful	Fine, soft or greying	Thin and coarse
Face	Large, rounded, full	Heart-shaped, chin sometimes pointed	Sharp features, angular or irregular
Eyes – size	Large, prominent	Average	Small, narrow or sunken
Eyes – lustre	Moist with thick eyelashes	Intense, sharp and penetrating. Can be red or bloodshot	Dry with thin lashes
Nose	Large, wide or rounded	Neat, straight, pointed, average in size	Small, long and narrow
Mouth	Large	Medium	Small
Lips	Big, full, velvety	Medium, red, soft	Thin, narrow, tight, may be dry or dark
Teeth	Large, straight, white with strong gums	Medium and yellowish	Irregular or protruding
Neck	Solid, thick	Average in proportion	Thin and long
Shoulders	Wide	Medium	Narrow
Hips	Wide	Medium	Narrow
Fingers	Wide, angular	Regular	Small and long
Nails	Smooth, large, shining and square	Soft, medium and pink	Rough, brittle or small
Feet	Large, wide	Medium	Small, narrow

Physiology

Sweat	Moderate to heavy with pleasant odour	Profuse with sharp odour	Minimal and odourless
Temperature – body	Cool and damp hands and feet	Warm, pink hands and feet	Cold and dry hands and feet
Temperature – preferences	Craves warmth	Loves coolness	Dislikes cold
Thirst	Scanty	Excessive	Variable
Appetite	Slow but steady	Good, excessive, unbearable	Variable, scanty
Taste preferences	Pungent, bitter, astringent and dry	Sweet, bitter, astringent, light and warm	Sweet, sour, salt and oily
Elimination – stool	Thick, oily, heavy and slow	Soft and well formed	Irregular or constipated. Dry, hard and dark
Elimination – urine	Profuse, infrequent	Normal but frequent	Little but frequent
Sleep	Heavy and prolonged	Short but sound	Light and interrupted
Speech	Slow, low, measured and may be laboured	Sharp, clear, precise and argumentative	Fast, talkative, interrupts
Physical activity	Lethargic	Moderate	Very active
Energy levels	Strong and sustained	Moderate and measured, lacks stamina	Short bursts and tires quickly
Walking	Slow, stable	Moderate and purposeful	Fast, short, quick steps

Emotions

Mind	Calm, slow	Aggressive, sharp and intelligent	Restless, active
Thinking	Steady and cannot be rushed	Precise, logical	Quick and creative with many ideas
Memory	Good long-term, takes time to learn	Good, quick	Poor long-term, good short-term
Decision making	Well thought out	Quick, decisive	Problematic
Beliefs and values	Not easily changed	Extremely strong convictions	Changes frequently
Creativity	In the area of business	Inventive and technical or scientific	Distinct and rich in ideas
Finances	Saves, thrifty	Methodical, spends on luxuries	Spends easily, can be wasteful
Work preferences	Caring	Intellectual	Creative
Lifestyle	Steady and regular	Busy, but plans to achieve much	Erratic
Relationships	Strong and loving	Jealous and possessive	Flirtatious and changing
Temperament:	**Tick all that apply to you**		
	Steady	Intense	Changeable
	Patient	Impatient	Sensitive
	Solicitous	Judgmental	Shy
	Lethargic	Ambitious	Nervous
	Self-satisfied	Competitive	Insecure
	Resilient	Practical	Intuitive
Do you like:			
	Stability	Self-development	Sun
	Quiet	Sports	Travel
	Business	Politics	Art
	Good food	Luxury	Esoteric subjects
Do you dislike:			
	Cold and damp	Heat and midday sun	Cold, wind and dryness

If you scored highest in the first column then you are a kapha dominant constitution.

If you scored highest in the middle column then you are a pitta dominant constitution.

If you scored highest in the last column then you are a vata dominant constitution.

Most people are a combination of the doshas rather than purely vata, pitta or kapha, with a dominance of one dosha.

Understanding your type

The following brief descriptions will help to confirm your personal constitution. Most people recognise a combination of doshas in their mental and physical characteristics so this is an opportunity to understand your own makeup in more detail.

The vata type

Vata types can be described as being cold, dry and irregular. According to traditional descriptions, vata people are generally either quite tall or quite short, with thin frames, flat chests and visible veins and muscle tendons. The skin is cold, rough, dry and cracked and they have prominent joints that are prone to cracking sounds. Their hands and feet are often cold.

Appetite and digestion in vata types tend to be variable and they crave sweet, sour and salty tastes. They like hot drinks, foods and weather. Urine production can be scanty and the faeces are dry, often giving rise to constipation. Their sleep may be disturbed and they will sleep less than other constitutional types.

Mentally, vata types may be quick to understand but also quick to forget. They are creative and active but are easily fatigued. They are very alert but can be restless and walk and talk quickly. In an unbalanced state, vata leads to feelings of being nervous, fearful and anxious with a tendency towards mental instability, low tolerance and will power.

Features of aggravated vata

- Pain, emaciation, dryness and degeneration
- Tremors, desire for heat and black discolouration on skin, around eyes, etc
- Loss of consciousness and impaired sense of perception
- Decrease in strength, weight loss and debility

- Constipation and flatulence
- Delusion, timidity, fear, grief, nervousness and confusion
- Diseases such as rheumatism, osteoarthritis and osteoporosis

Causes of vata imbalance

- Irregular lifestyle
- Sudden changes in life, season or environment
- Physical or mental exhaustion
- Advanced stages of addictions
- A diet including cold, raw or dried foods; too much bitter, astringent or spicy food
- Being on irregular or stringent diets
- Suffering from grief, fear, or unexpected shocks
- Exposure to cold, dry and windy weather
- Ignoring the body's natural urges
- Travelling, especially flying
- Erratic sleep patterns

The pitta type

Pitta types can be described as being hot, oily and irritable. According to traditional descriptions these types are of medium height, weight and body frame with moderate muscle development. Complexion may be coppery, yellowish or fair compared to others in the same ethnic group and they may suffer from moles or freckles. Skin tends to be soft, warm and less wrinkled than vata skin. Hair can be thin and silky with a tendency for thinning or premature greying. Any Caucasians with red or fair hair have an element of pitta. Eyes can be intense, slightly reddish and moist.

Pitta types have a good digestion and strong appetite and can usually consume large quantities of food and drink. They crave sweet, bitter and astringent tastes and enjoy cooling foods and drinks. There is a tendency towards slightly higher body temperature and excessive perspiration with warm hands and feet. Pitta types do not tolerate heat or sunlight very well.

Mentally pitta people are intelligent, sharp with good speaking skills and comprehension. In an imbalanced state they can tend towards fiery emotions such as hate, anger and jealousy. Pittas are ambitious types and generally make good leaders.

Features of aggravated pitta

- Burning sensation, increase in temperature, thirst and desire for cold comforts
- Yellow discolouration of skin, eyes etc and bitter taste in mouth
- Fatigue and fainting
- Impaired digestion and disrupted sleep
- Anger and aggression

Causes of pitta imbalance

- Reacting to stress with suppressed anger, frustration and resentment
- Placing excessive demands and not tolerating wasted time
- Being exposed to many high-pressure situations or to violent stimuli
- Eating too much hot, spicy, oily, fried, salty, fermented food or alcohol
- Being exposed to hot, humid weather, impure food and water
- Bad sunburn or heat exhaustion

The kapha type

Kapha types can be described as being cold, wet and stable. According to traditional descriptions kapha people are generally well developed physically with thick skin and muscle, broad chests but with a tendency to carry excess weight. Complexion tends to be fair and bright with skin that is soft, lustrous, oily, but cold and pale when compared with those of the same ethnic group. The eyes can be dark or blue and the white part clear, large and very white.

Digestion for kapha types can be slow but very regular with a requirement for less intake of food and a craving for pungent, bitter and astringent foods. Their sleep tends to be long and deep and they have excellent stamina.

Mentally, kapha types tend to be tolerant, calm and forgiving, but in an imbalanced state can show traits of greed, attachment, envy and possessiveness. They can also tend towards lethargy and inaction. Comprehension, speech and movement can be slow but long-term memory is excellent.

Features of aggravated kapha

- Heaviness, coldness and obstruction of channels
- Fatigue, fainting and sleepiness

- Weak digestive capacity, excess salivation and nausea
- Whitish discoloration and itching of skin or mucus membranes
- Obesity and weight gain
- Difficulty in breathing and cough

Causes of kapha imbalance

- Remaining sedentary for a long time
- Overindulgence in a rich diet. Excessive fat, chocolate, sweet, salty and sour foods
- Feeling too contented, lacking impetus for growth, reluctance to change
- Eating frequently. Eating before the previous meal is digested. Eating too many snacks
- Overeating
- Oversleeping
- Lack of physical and mental work. Lack of exercise
- Exposure to cold, moist weather

The terms 'dry', 'oily', etc are all traditional Ayurvedic descriptions of constitutional types and may at first sound a little strange. In general terms they refer to physical and functional characteristics. For example, vata types are considered dry. Physically, this may manifest in dry skin, hair and nails. Functionally, this dryness can result in lack of lubrication for efficient digestion and cause conditions such as constipation. Kapha types on the other hand are naturally oily. This may manifest in oily skin or greasy hair. It provides natural lubrication for all mucus membranes, but in excess, mucus being a form of kapha, can cause conditions such as congestion in the upper respiratory tract or stools. Try and apply the descriptions in the broadest sense to your own physical, functional and mental characteristics.

Using constitution skilfully

Remember that your constitution represents your preferences and natural inclinations and is not intended to stereotype you. It is simply to help you to better understand yourself and how to actively manage the things that affect your health such as food, activities and thinking styles. Under Skilful Activity we will discuss in detail how to best use the natural cyclical process to your advantage. The doshas respond in unique ways to different foods and we will discuss this in some detail under Skilful Eating. Knowing your constitution enables you to manage your relationships with others who may be of a different constitutional type. We will take a look at using constitution in the workplace, helping you to manage your stress levels and also the relationships with your colleagues.

If it is accurate, your constitution is a reflection of you and your natural preferences. There is no right or wrong in these preferences and one constitution is no better than another, only different. These differences between constitutional types can be extremely valuable and if used skilfully will help you to recognise your own and other's natural strengths. These differences may manifest in many ways: the areas on which individuals like to focus their attention, the way that they communicate or absorb information, the way that they respond to the environment and the lifestyle they prefer to adopt. Therefore, constitution helps to:

- Improve your health and energy levels through the skilful use of food, activity and thinking
- Identify mental and physical inclinations that come most naturally to you
- Recognise and strengthen opposite inclinations that may be weak
- Improve the quality and productivity of your relationship with others.

one

skilful eating

Skilful eating is about gaining mastery of our eating habits to provide us with supercharged energy and overall health.

In Ayurveda, man is considered to be literally that which he eats; physically, mentally and energetically. So, if food is the main source of energy for our body and mind, does that mean we eat only the food that is most beneficial for our bodies in quantities for optimum functioning? Unfortunately, not in most cases! We have a complex relationship with food and our eating choices are often driven more by our emotions than our functional needs. We *are* going to discuss balancing our diet and eating the foods appropriate for your constitution, but first we must address our emotional relationship with food. This is because we are looking to make permanent changes in our behaviour. Many of us use food to replace emotional deficits elsewhere in our life, or as a result of conditioned behaviour that does not necessarily give us the things we say we want. Part of building the framework for a skilful eating plan is to lay solid emotional foundations.

Ayurveda takes a slightly different approach to food than conventional diet and nutrition. Here we will explore the energetics of food, but also the *when*, *how* and *why* of eating. It will require you to separate your emotional cravings from your true needs. This is not about turning the eating experience into a dull, mechanical process – quite the opposite in fact. When we are truly in control of our eating habits, as with all other aspects of our life, our experiences are expansive and joyful, allowing us to reflect the passion of one of life's wonderful gifts. Once you are in touch with your body, you will delight in eating the things that your body loves, and which nourish you not only physically, but also emotionally and mentally.

Our body is continually giving us signals about what is beneficial and what is not. Many of us have lost touch with these messages and our eating reflects our conditioned habits rather than our natural intuitive state.

Skilful Eating is not about prescribing a list of dos and don'ts. It is about reconnecting with this most natural, intuitive state. As we described earlier, we will concentrate on the positive by getting back in touch with our bodies. But it is also useful to understand our current limiting behaviour and explore the processes that drive our relationship with food.

Understanding your food history

Observe young children and babies. They are very in touch with what their bodies need; they will eat when they are hungry and only in the amounts that they require. Even breast milk, which is nectar for most infants, will be refused if the child has consumed enough. So we enter this life programmed to be in touch with our most fundamental needs – it is only when this intuition is replaced through other conditioned responses that we lose touch.

I grew up in an environment that had a healthy attitude to food. However, no matter what the level of awareness of your upbringing, you unwittingly absorb the experiences and outlook of those most influential around you. In most cases this is our parents or carers. My father was raised after the Second World War in a family with ten children. Food during this period was scarce and meal times were less about diet and nutrition than about survival. For him, leaving the dinner table feeling stuffed was a luxury that did not happen very often. This generated a strong connection between security and comfort and having a full stomach. This is a powerful emotional association and one that is almost inevitably passed through to the next generation. Many of us probably recognise the cries around the dinner table about eating everything on your dinner plate regardless of how hungry you are. Wasted food is punished and an empty plate is rewarded. (This is meant as a non-critical observation, about an ethic of a generation who rightly recognised the value of food and expressed it the best way that they could).

So, even when the threat of food being a scarce commodity has disappeared, this system of reward and punishment perpetuates a feeling of comfort associated with a full stomach. When our children have behaved in a way that we approve of, we very often demonstrate this approval by rewarding them with a sugary snack. So it is not surprising that we have a generation of adults for whom acceptance, approval, comfort and love are directly associated with eating large amounts and with high-sugar foods.

If you don't know it already, determine your own personal food history. This understanding will help to raise your awareness of how you use food on an emotional level and will help you to break unwanted patterns.

Alongside our childhood influences, there will be other significant events in our life that shape our expression of emotion through our relationship with food. I have known people with eating disorders who have taken their relationship with food to a point where it is life-threatening. Traumatic events are often overwhelming and, in contrast, food can seem to be one of the few things we can control. This attempt at controlling emotions through eating habits, however, often has the opposite effect: our behaviour is so restrictive and limiting that the food is really in control of us. To be truly free of these patterns we need to fully understand our own personal history with food, and the subtle emotional associations we have made that drive our habits. Food does not enter our body by accident, but by choice. We need to understand the motivation behind these choices.

Take a few minutes to answer the following questions:

What are your earliest or most powerful food experiences?

● What was the food culture like when you were young?

● Was there a reward and punishment system in operation?

● How did that work? Did you have to eat everything? Was not eating your veg punished?

● How did the reward system work and what were you rewarded with?

● Which parent or carer provided the discipline and what is their food history?

Do you recognise any patterns in your eating?

● Are there particular occasions when you overeat or eat particular things? For example, when you are stressed or upset.

● How do you reward yourself?

● How do you feel after eating? For example, satisfied, guilty, energised.

What are the most important changes you would like to make to your eating experiences?

Recognising our influences and the resulting associations is a good starting point for making changes. However, rather than breaking old associations, the most powerful way of effecting change is to make new ones. The most positive connections we can make are those associated with our inherent functional needs and our fundamental nature. As far as food is concerned, this means getting back in touch with your body. This is exactly what we will do in this section using awareness exercises, but first let's have a look at some basic principles of Ayurveda. These will help us to make lasting changes.

The Ayurvedic view of food

Ayurveda asserts that all substances have the potential to be nutritious or poisonous depending upon their application. Even the purest of foods can become harmful if used inappropriately, by certain constitutions or at the wrong time. What is nourishing for one person can result in imbalance, and ultimately in illness, for another.

The phrase, 'Man is what he eats' originated with Ayurveda and is taken very literally. Our body tissues are created from the substances we put in our mouths. But the issue isn't just what we eat, it is about how well that food is absorbed through our digestive system. The quality of our digestion is the key factor in the transformation of food either into healthy tissues, waste or toxins. The transformation of food into energetic and physical components of the body is influenced not only by what we eat, but also when, where and how we eat. So, Ayurveda takes an integrated view of our eating experience. It views food from an energetic, rather than a molecular point of view and considers actions within the body in relation to the balance of doshas rather than in terms of purely physical effects. Also, the pattern and timing of your eating are as important as what you eat and the effect of this upon your personal constitution. This approach may at first seem a little complicated, but you will find that it's actually very simple and powerful. Its practicality will be revealed later when we look at how to achieve the perfectly balanced diet.

The three energies

To truly understand how this system of energetics works, we need to understand a number of key concepts in Ayurveda that underpin the system and how we can use them in a practical way. The three doshas, vata, pitta and kapha, each have a subtle counterpart called, respectively, prana, agni and ojas. These are vital forces in our body that, when in perfect balance, will provide fantastic energy levels and glowing health.

Agni

The principle of fire in the universe and in our body is called agni. It is not simply fire in the elemental sense; it is a subtle energy, related to pitta dosha and responsible for all transformation processes in the body. These include the assimilation of thoughts and ideas that produces understanding as well as the transformation of food, via digestion, into our body tissues. We will use it in the sense of digestive fire. Both Ayurveda and yoga are about the understanding of agni. Disease in Ayurveda is described in terms of the poor functioning of agni. Treatment often centres on rekindling this fire so that it acts efficiently. Its function directly affects the quality of our body tissues, such as the skin, and our energy levels. It not only influences physical health, but also our intellectual processes of perception and understanding. Agni is affected directly by what we eat just as fuel added to a fire can produce a strong flame or douse it all together. Agni has natural peaks throughout the day. These high points in its cycle produce the optimum periods of the day for eating. All of our eating habits can be described in relation to their effect upon agni.

Ojas

Ojas is kapha dosha in its purest form and its abundance in the body is as a result of pure and efficient digestion. Ojas is considered to be the ultimate product of this transformational process and helps to support tissues that are vital and healthy. Ojas can be related to our natural immunity and gives us a natural radiance and glow, enabling us to fight off most diseases. Although ojas permeates all healthy body tissue, its seat is in the area of the heart, as with kapha dosha. By the consumption of food that is appropriate for our body, the efficient functioning of agni is supported and the vital energy of ojas generated.

Prana

Prana is the most sublime form of vata dosha and supports our most dynamic functions, helping to efficiently coordinate our breath, senses and higher states of consciousness. It is actively managed through the appropriate intake of food, Ayurvedic therapies and the practice of yoga, particularly breathing exercises.

So, as with the three doshas, the subtle energy forces of agni, ojas and prana are completely interdependent on each other. Prana is the mobilising force for all functions in the body and mind, supporting the efficient transformation process of agni. When these two energies are working in harmony, the production of ojas is the result. Only with an abundance of ojas can the function of agni and prana be assured. Likewise, only through the aware management of the three pillars of eating, activity and thinking can these subtle energies work actively for our optimum health.

The Transformation of Food

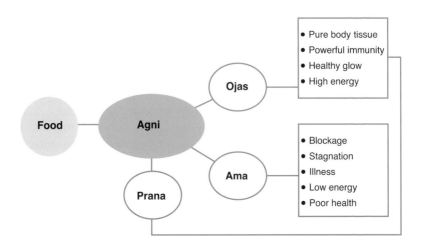

Ama

When disharmony exists between the three energies and the three doshas, our internal processes are not able to produce pure body tissues or optimum levels of energy. Food that does not properly transform into healthy tissues or natural waste becomes a toxin in the body called ama. It is considered to be a waxy substance, produced as a result of impaired agni and can spread anywhere in the system resulting in blockage, stagnation and ill health. Often the first line of action in Ayurvedic treatment of disease is to rid the body of ama. Any detoxification treatment will help to eliminate ama and create a lighter, more energetic feel.

These are not just abstract concepts. An understanding of these energy forces helps us to balance them through careful management of the doshas, and so create practical results. Because we are trying to balance subtle energies in the body, Ayurveda takes a completely integrated approach to eating. Here we will consider the nature of the food we eat, how it interacts with our personal constitution and how the amount, place and nature of our eating habits affect our health. This is described under the *Ayurvedic discipline of balanced eating* and provides some powerful advice for our use of food. By following this approach, you will balance the subtle energies of agni, ojas and prana.

The Ayurvedic Discipline of Balanced Eating

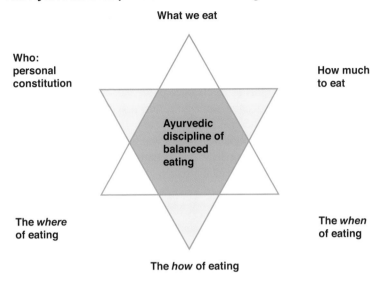

How **much** to eat

We've already implied that through our social conditioning we tend to overeat. Yogis say that to significantly increase our life span we should halve the amount of food we eat! More recently, animal studies have shown that a 30 per cent reduction in food intake halted the growth of tumours in the animals, and doubled their life expectancy. So, eating only as much as our body truly needs is a skill worth developing. According to the principles of yoga, if you are eating a healthy amount, your stomach is half filled by the food eaten and one quarter filled with fluid. The rest is empty space that allows efficient digestion to occur. With some practice it is possible to become sensitive to these quantities.

Ideal Stomach Contents After a Meal

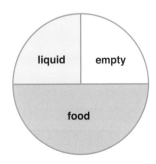

Generally speaking, we are only consciously aware of any body part when there is a problem with it. For example, only when we have a headache do we become consciously aware of the head – during most other times we don't even think about it. If you become aware of a heaviness in your stomach as you are eating, then you have probably already eaten too much. This feeling is caused by the stretch receptors around your stomach signalling strain. Use this as a reference point and work backwards from this amount of food and, at the same time, tune in with the feelings you are experiencing. With practice you will be able to judge the optimum amounts for your body. Here's a simple test: when you walk away from the dinner table you should be feeling light and energised, not bloated, heavy or lethargic. Always try to finish eating on a high.

Eating like a child

Never eat unless you are hungry. Sounds simple, but how often do we eat out of habit, because others are eating, or to gain a feeling of comfort or reward from the consumption of certain foods? We mentioned earlier that children, before they are conditioned to behave otherwise, generally eat only when they are hungry. This is because they are paying attention to their bodies. To help get back in tune with these messages try to get used to assessing your hunger before you eat anything. On a scale of 1 – 10, where 10 is ravenously hungry, judge the strength of your hunger. If it is between 1 and 5, then go and do something else to distract you from your craving. Anything between 6 and 10 probably means your body is in need of some nourishment, so eat and enjoy!

The **when** of eating

Natural cycles are something we will also discuss in the next section, Skilful Activity, but they're worth mentioning here because the timing of *when* we eat is almost as important as *what* we eat.

Due to a lack of awareness of our natural energetic cycles, many people get into a cycle of eating that can be destructive to their energy levels and health. We live busy lifestyles that often push our eating habits into the periods of the day where we can practically fit them. This may not always be the best time for our bodies.

Many people tend to eat late in the evening and often close to bedtime. They get up in the morning have a quick breakfast, or miss it altogether – often not feeling hungry because they have not finished digesting the meal from the previous evening. Having missed breakfast, they then perhaps drink some tea or coffee around mid morning, and eat a snack to boost blood sugar levels and keep them going. Lunch is often something light, like a sandwich at the desk, because they've already been eating and are under pressure. Another snack and a coffee in the afternoon props up flagging energy until the evening meal. Because of the afternoon snack most are not hungry until later in the evening when the largest meal of the day is eaten and the downward energy cycle begins again.

This cycle ensures that we are dictated to by external circumstances rather than by bodily needs and usually means we are one step behind the amount of energy we need for our daily activities. Ayurveda defines a number of energetic cycles that operate throughout our day, and describes how to work with them so as to maximise our energy levels.

Daily cycles

The day is broken into six cycles where one of the three doshas is more active.

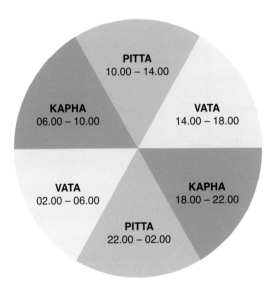

If we are smart, we can align certain daily activities to coincide with these periods to counteract or balance certain forces. This requires us to know a little about the functions of the three doshas, the things that they are responsible for and also our own constitution.

Kapha period: 06.00 – 10.00

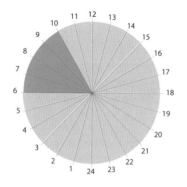

Key kapha activities:

- Ideal time for the 15-minute routine of yoga, breathing and visualisation (see Skilful Activity section)

- Complete the morning daily routine described in the Skilful Activity section

- Eat light and easily digestible food.

Recall that kapha is a heavy, grounded energy force and during this period you may experience a heavy or sluggish feeling. Kapha is also responsible for sleep. To make a smooth transition from the resting to the active period of the day, we need to shake off some of the heavy kapha influences. To do this, the following should be applied.

Eat light, easily digestible food which allows your body to make a smooth transition from sleeping to waking and your agni to reach its peak. As kapha is a cold energy, a glass of warm water is a good first thing to hit your stomach. It counteracts kapha and stimulates agni, particularly if a squeeze of lemon or lime is added. Breakfast is important as it will give you the energy to reach lunchtime. Counteract this heaviness of kapha by eating light. Fruit is very light to digest and is a perfect, natural way to start your day. We will discuss which fruits and other food substances are suitable for which constitutions a little later. A heavy breakfast will tend to aggravate kapha dosha and may cause heaviness, bloating and lethargy.

Pitta period 10.00 – 14.00

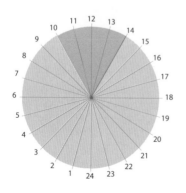

Key pitta activities:

- Eat the main meal of the day

- Eat the food appropriate for your constitution in the optimum quantities

- Great time of the day for complex problem solving and intellectual activities.

We've already established that pitta is directly related to agni and that agni is responsible for all of our transformational processes, particularly digestion. This is the period of the day when agni is at its peak and our digestive energy is very high. This means that ideally, our main meal of the day should be eaten during this period.

I can hear the cries of despair and dissent this suggestion will cause. On every workshop that I run, people react by calling this either difficult or impossible. But before deciding on this, let's look a little more closely at what it means.

When we consider our main meal, it must be in the context of our personal constitution and the balancing of this meal against our other meals that day. The foods that are heavier or more difficult to digest should be eaten during this period. Any animal proteins, for example, should be consumed at this time of the day. We've already discussed the quantities that are appropriate, so don't form an image of Desperate Dan size plates of cow pie here! It's beneficial to eat a meal that is warm and moist that includes all six tastes (as described later), rather than a quick sandwich and packet of crisps. Also, if the profile of our breakfast is appropriate, light and early, then it should be well on its way to being digested and we should be feeling a strong hunger. So you should be ready for a proper meal.

Also, we are often constrained by our working lives. Yet this should not necessarily mean that this dictates our energy levels and our health. You will have to decide where your health sits in your list of priorities and perhaps challenge some of the habits built around your working day. This may mean preparing food and bringing it into work, eating somewhere else, or simply taking the lunch break properly away from your desk. This is your choice. As far as your body is concerned, this is the optimum time to eat your main meal. In consultations I have often achieved amazing improvements in people's energy and health by simply changing the profile of their daily eating habits. Usually, before we even significantly change their diet, I will adjust their daily routine to the one described here and, within a couple of weeks, noticeable improvements in energy and vitality are achieved.

Often people fear that if a larger meal is eaten at lunch, then they will feel heavy and sluggish. However, if the appropriate food has been eaten for your constitution, and in the optimum amount, then this sense of heaviness should be avoided. You should finish your meal with a sense of lightness and a level of energy that will comfortably take you through to your evening meal.

Vata period 14.00 – 18.00

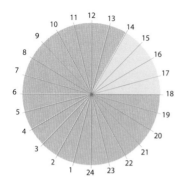

Key vata activities:

- Avoid stimulants such as tea, coffee or refined sugar

- Avoid snacking before your lunch has digested and too close to the evening meal

- Consume warm drinks such as herb or fruit teas

- Snack on fresh or dried fruit if absolutely necessary.

Recall that vata dosha is light, dynamic and changeable. If you have eaten appropriately over lunch, then this feeling of lightness and energy should be experienced. This is often the time of the day we tend to suffer an afternoon dip in energy. This may be because we have eaten a quick sandwich on the run, coupled with a sugary snack, which gives us a short boost but does not last long. However, if we have followed some of the rules of skilful eating, our body will still be digesting our lunch time meal and won't need an energy top-up. One of the advantages of taking our main meal in the middle of the day is that our body then has the active hours of the afternoon to digest and assimilate the food. This will give us a much more balanced energy profile in the afternoon and will easily sustain us until our evening meal.

Vata is also cold and dry in nature and this may be counteracted by consuming a hot drink. Stimulants such as tea or coffee should be avoided as vata is already a highly stimulated energy force. Drink an alternative such as fruit or herb tea instead. Something like fresh ginger tea would be perfect as the ginger in hot water will balance the cold vata energy.

Also, many people often mistake their body's need for fluid as a hunger pang. If you think you are hungry during this period, then have a drink first and then do the hunger test once more. If you really cannot do without something to eat during this period, then snack on a piece of fruit – the sweetness will balance vata and digestion will most likely be complete before the evening meal.

Kapha period 18.00 – 22.00

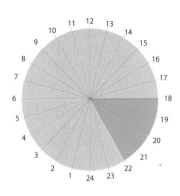

Key kapha activities:

- Eat light and early – ideally before 20.00

- Maintain the ritual of an evening meal, but without the difficult-to-digest animal proteins

- Drink a little hot water or milk before going to bed

- Avoid daytime sleep

- Another good period for exercise.

This is the second kapha peak of the day and is the period when most people eat an evening meal. We've already established that our main meal of the day should have been a number of hours ago during the pitta period. This does not mean that we do not have a meal in the evening, only that the profile reflects the predominant kapha energy as well as what has been eaten before.

The heavy kapha energy should again be countered by lighter eating to aid this potentially sluggish period. Lightness essentially refers to those substances that we find easy to digest. Avoid animal proteins if you can, ideally making the meal vegetarian. Also, it is beneficial to have finished eating before about 20.00, leaving at least two or three hours before you go to bed. Eating before sleep leads to poorly digested food and the formation of ama. The only exception is the consumption of warm water or milk as this helps to flush toxins and aids sleep.

Pitta period 22.00 – 02.00

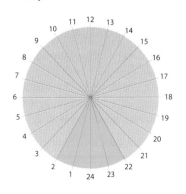

Key pitta activities:

- Avoid eating

- Sleep!

This pitta period is good for assimilating and transforming the day's intake of food. If you are up and active during this period then it is the pitta energy that often drives your craving for a midnight snack. The late night take-away industry has unknowingly built a successful trade on the pitta energy peak in this period! Avoid eating altogether unless you are working shifts.

Vata period 02.00 – 06.00

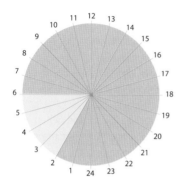

Key vata activities:

- Ideal time to rise with the sun and practise the dynamic yoga routine
- Ideal time to eliminate bodily waste.

In yoga philosophy the period, just before the sun rises, is the ideal time to get up! It is called *Brahma Muhurta* and waking is aided by the light energetic nature of vata. It is also the best time for our natural elimination processes to take place as vata dosha is responsible for all excretory functions in the body. This having been said, most people tend to rise during the following kapha period and as a result must counter its heavy energy as described earlier.

The skilful cycle

This is a complete cycle, and you will find that once in the routine, a certain momentum is achieved. Our body is cyclical in nature, but it may be that the cycle you currently practise is dictated by external circumstances and does not provide you with your optimum levels of energy. The above skilful cycle follows your body's natural rhythms and with a little practice will fall naturally into place. For example, if you have eaten early and light the night before, your sleep is better and you feel lighter and more refreshed in the morning. Eating light during the morning kapha period gives you more energy and a strong feeling of hunger for the afternoon meal. The afternoon pitta period will help to digest your main meal of the day and give you enough energy to get to the evening meal without a need to snack.

However, this continuous cycle is more important than the absolute times given. Experiment with your own body and the way you can fit the routine into your own life. Once you do drop into a routine, I guarantee that you will feel the benefits in energy and well-being.

Summary of Key Skills

02.00 – 06.00 Vata period
Key elimination period

Do:
- Consider rising with the sun

Avoid:
- The suppression of any natural elimination urges

06.00 – 10.00 Kapha period
Do:
- Get your body moving – complete the 15-minute routine of yoga, breathing and visualisation
- Complete the morning routine described later
- Eat a light, energetic breakfast

Avoid:
- Anything heavy, artificially sweet or difficult to digest

10.00 – 14.00 Pitta period
Key appropriation period

Do:
- Eat main meal of the day in line with Skilful Principles

Avoid:
- Overeating, anything too spicy or oily

14.00 – 18.00 Vata period
Do:
- Consume plenty of liquids particularly warm herb or fruit teas

Avoid:
- Stimulants such as tea, coffee or refined sugars
- Snacking before lunch has been digested and too close to the evening meal

18.00 – 22.00 Kapha period
Do:
- Eat light and early – ideally before 20.00
- Maintain the ritual of an evening meal but without the difficult-to-digest animal proteins
- Consider some exercise or yoga
- Drink a little hot water or milk before bed

Avoid:
- Daytime sleep!

22.00 – 02.00 Pitta period
Key assimilation period

Do:
- Sleep and allow the body's natural transformation processes to absorb the benefits of the day's food and exercise

Avoid:
- Eating anything!

Keeping a Food and Activity Diary

Awareness of your own body rhythms and your reactions to food, pressure and other daily stimuli are key pieces of information. Once you are aware of them you can adjust your activity and behaviour to make the most of them.

This exercise is aimed at making you body-aware. For two weeks keep a food and activity diary. Record what and when you eat, and the effects it has upon your energy levels and feeling of well-being. Also, be aware of the emotional associations you identified in the section on your food history. In addition, record the physical activity you undertake – include walking as well as any exercise or yoga you practise. Notice the effect on your digestion, energy and sleeping. Be honest with yourself! Although this is a simple exercise, it can be very powerful in spotting patterns in your habits that may actually be working against your best interests.

Copy the table opposite and record your activities daily for at least two weeks:

Example Food and Activity Diary

Date:

Breakfast:
07.00 – 1 Toast with butter and jam

Lunch:
12.30 – Tuna sandwich, crisps and a chocolate bar

Evening meal:
20.00 – Spaghetti bolognaise, ice cream and 2 glasses of wine

Snacks:
10.00 – Yogurt and biscuit
15.00 – Jam doughnut and coffee

Drinks:	Tea: 5	Coffee: 1	Water: 1ltr
	Herbal: 0	Other: 2 glasses wine	

Energy levels/emotions:
● Heavy and not hungry on waking
● Energy dip in afternoon – feeling tired and stressed (had a snack and coffee, felt better at first, but didn't last long!)
● Felt better after evening yoga – more light and relaxed (also more hungry)

Exercise:
● Walk to station – 10 min
● 15 min yoga and breathing at 18.00

General comments:
● Noticed I'm not very hungry around lunch or dinner because of snacks
● Felt much more hungry after exercise in evening
● Fell asleep in chair after evening meal and wine!
● Will try and do a little yoga in the morning

Food and Activity Diary

Date:

Breakfast:

Lunch:

Evening meal:

Snacks:

Drinks: **Tea:** ☐   **Coffee:** ☐   **Water:** ☐

Herbal: ☐   **Other:** ☐

Energy levels/emotions:

Exercise:

General comments:

Being more in touch with these rhythms is an important part of living skilfully. Once you feel this increased connection you will have a better idea of what works for you and what things will increase your state of health. It may not eliminate the external factors that may be causing stress in your life, but it will give you greater resources to cope. Having a routine in life is healthy. Such anchors help us to cope with stressful situations and give some certainty and regularity to circumstances that otherwise may be outside our control. If we can develop anchors that follow our natural cycles, we find that we also have nature on our side.

Once you have kept your food and activity diary for a two-week period, change your routine to reflect the skilful eating cycle for another period of two weeks. It may feel a little uncomfortable at first to alter your fundamental eating habits, but if necessary force the routine initially. All change processes feel uncomfortable at first! Continue to keep your food and activity diary over this period and particularly note any changes to your energy, mood or sense of well-being. If the new cycle works for you then you will not need any further encouragement to continue!

The **how** of eating

Because Ayurveda is based upon a system of energetics, how we eat and our awareness during the consumption of our food are very important. Eating should be a joyful experience, one where we employ our senses and become engaged in the colours, smells and textures. We must also be aware of the more subtle effects that food has on our body and be aware of the digestive process as a whole.

Assessing your digestion:

Use this simple questionnaire to assess the current state of your digestion. Place a tick in any box that applies to you:

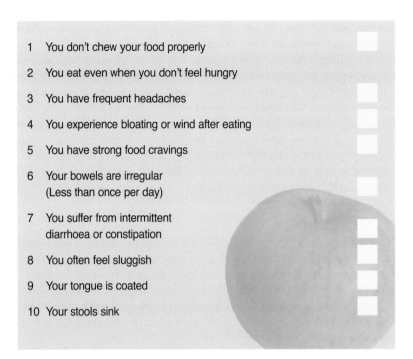

1   You don't chew your food properly

2   You eat even when you don't feel hungry

3   You have frequent headaches

4   You experience bloating or wind after eating

5   You have strong food cravings

6   Your bowels are irregular
    (Less than once per day)

7   You suffer from intermittent
    diarrhoea or constipation

8   You often feel sluggish

9   Your tongue is coated

10 Your stools sink

If you ticked five or more boxes, then it is likely you are suffering from poor digestion and it needs some support through your eating habits.

Improving awareness of digestion

Digestion is a process that starts with consumption and ends with either the absorption of nutrients into the body, the elimination of waste, or (if we don't get things right) the deposit of toxins in our body in the form of ama. The digestive tract, or *koshta* in Ayurveda, is considered to be outside of the body as it is a closed tube with one end at the mouth and the other at the anus. Food enters at one end and exits at the other with the useful bits being absorbed along the way. If we are to truly get in touch with our body, we need to be aware of each stage of this process and understand the messages we are sent.

Our eating experience starts before we put food into our mouths. The sights and smells of food all produce powerful emotional and physical reactions that effectively prepare our body for digesting the incoming food. We react with natural delight at the colours and aromas of many foods, which produce a strong natural desire to eat as well as responses such as salivation. This stimulation of our senses is part of the joy of eating, but also an active ingredient in our downfall. We live in a sense-driven society and the instant satisfaction of how something looks, smells and tastes, as well as the image associated with certain foods, influences our eating choices more than anything else. This becomes a problem only if we are passive participants in this sensory experience. When we are totally engaged with this important, but superficial stimulation of our senses, we are very often disengaged from the consequent results further along the digestive process. The result, of course, is that we often choose food that looks, smells and tastes good, but is destructive to our body. This disconnection means that the very mechanism that is designed to aid our digestion works against us. The key to solving this is to be aware of the entire eating experience, not just the bit that ends when we swallow.

Sensory awareness exercise

This exercise is to get you back in touch with your internal environment through the active engagement of your senses. There is a big difference between passive stimulation and active involvement with our senses. Sitting and watching the television does not necessarily require an engagement of the mind, even though our senses may be stimulated. As with much of our inherent physical and mental equipment, the use of our senses today falls very short of their full capacity.

Hearing

Next time you sit down to eat a meal, take a few minutes to tune in to your senses. Gently close your eyes and for a few seconds focus on your breath, allowing yourself to relax. By closing your eyes you are eliminating visual stimulation, which for many is their most influential sense. Bring your awareness inside your body and you will hear the sound of your breath and perhaps the pulse of your heartbeat. Be aware of yourself as the centre of the experience. Tune into your hearing and gradually move the radius outward to pick up the sounds going on around you, separating out the layers. The sounds close by may seem impossible to get beyond at first, but you will find you can tune in and out. Judge where the sounds are coming from – not only the direction, but also the distance. The layers are not only to do with proximity, they also involve intensity. There may be constant background noises that, because of their repetitive nature, you had naturally tuned out. It may be the sound of the wind in the trees or perhaps other sounds that you had completely missed.

Smell

Once you have gathered as much information as you can through your hearing, switch your attention to the smells around you. Carry out much the same exercise as with your hearing. Centre yourself first and be aware of your own personal odour. This may be your scent or deodorant, or perhaps the solution you wash your clothes in. Again, move your sensory radius outwards and detect what you can, concentrating fully on your sense of smell, eliminating all other senses.

Touch

Next, turn your attention to your sense of touch. You may find this is subtler than the other senses. Again, start by calibrating your experience and be aware of your own skin. Detect the temperature and any other sensations that you judge to be coming from within. Turn your attention then to any external stimuli – you may feel the radiation of the sun through the window, or a breeze. You should feel the difference between those areas of your skin that are exposed and those that are covered with clothes. Explore the differences and dwell on the subtleties.

Vision

With your eyes still closed put all of your sensory information together. Look at the darkness behind your eyes and then open them. You may be startled at first by the intensity of the light and the colours. Verify the mental picture you had painted. Seek out the sounds and the smells and judge the direction and distance of the source. Spend time now taking in the scene around you. Again look beyond the obvious stimulation and concentrate on the layers. Deliberately look for the things you would normally miss.

Concentrate on the micro without losing how it fits with the macro. You may at first find this a superficial exercise, but done thoroughly it can be exhausting. As we are taking in information continually, we do this sub-consciously, almost as a habit. Bringing this to a conscious level takes effort.

Taste

Now you are ready to eat. Notice the colours of your food and the smells. Centre your sense of taste by being aware of any residual tastes in your mouth. Many cultures eat with the hand. This puts them in direct contact with their food and signals its temperature to their body, thereby allowing it to prepare. When you put your food in your mouth, increase the time that it is there and chew slowly and carefully. Our digestion actually starts in our mouth and chewing reduces the load on our stomach by breaking down the food and providing greater surface area for your gastric juices to work on. The chemical breakdown also begins here. Satisfaction signals are sent to your brain if the residence time in your mouth is long enough. Look for the layers of taste and, if you have not cooked the food yourself, try and determine what it contains, the spices, herbs and oil it was cooked in.

Ayurveda describes six tastes that are important from an energetic point of view. Try to isolate the tastes in your mouth and tune into the energetic effect they have on your body.

When you swallow, be aware of the passage of food into your stomach. Our stomach and small intestines are the seat of agni, the digestive fire. There is a balance of acid in the stomach and alkali in the small intestine that is important to good digestion. The acid breaks down the food particles and if this has not been done efficiently (through lack of chewing, or eating too quickly) more acid than alkali will be produced. This causes imbalance and indigestion. The balance can also be upset by eating food that is too acidic in nature (such as citrus fruits, vinegar, wine, spicy food and fried food). This over-stimulates agni and can cause ama to be formed. Be aware of how the food sits in your stomach. Do the quantity check that we described earlier – can you feel the stretch receptors around your stomach registering yet?

Practise this at each meal for one week and notice the difference in awareness of your eating experience. Although it is described here as an exercise, try to develop it as a life habit.

Elimination

Some of the above internal processes can be subtle and not so easy to detect. However, one good indicator of our digestive efficiency lies with our elimination processes. I'm sorry to bring this up, but what comes out of our body is key to understanding what is going on inside. If healthy, our passing of stools and urine should be regular and easy. Our stools should be soft, like a ripe banana, without obnoxious odour and generally produced at least once a day – although there will of course be differences between the constitutions. Vata types are very dry and can suffer from irregularity and constipation if not careful. Pitta types are fluid in nature but can suffer from diarrhoea or burning when passing stools when in an unbalanced state. Kapha types are oily in nature so should eliminate easily but, as their digestion often works a little slower than the other types, the frequency may be slightly lower. In general, anything from three times a day to once every three days can be considered normal, based upon your constitution. Regularity is much more important than frequency. Don't resist the urge to defecate or urinate as this will cause vata imbalance.

The frequency of urination also varies greatly but, if you are following the other Skilful Eating tips and drinking enough water, you should be emptying your bladder roughly once every two hours.

Being aware of the entire digestive process is an important skill to develop as it allows us to understand the consequences of our eating habits. Being acutely aware of how we eat our food allows us to make these connections and make better-informed eating choices.

To be sure that you are absorbing the optimum amount from your food, it is worth checking how long your food takes to pass through your system. You can do this by eating sweet corn, which will be seen in your stools on elimination. Again, the transit time will vary depending upon constitution, but around 24 hours is an optimum indicator. If it is less than 12 hours, or there is undigested food in your stools, you are probably not absorbing the right amount of nutrients from your food and should get it checked out by a qualified health practitioner.

The **where** of eating

Ayurveda considers that we absorb the energy of our surroundings when we eat, as well as the energy of the food and the person who cooks it. By taking time over the eating process, relaxing, chewing properly and being aware, you'll make an amazing difference to your eating experience. Try to put the ceremony back into your eating habits. When I was growing up, meal times were generally a social affair with the family sat around the dinner table. In this way, eating became much more than simply a refuelling exercise.

Because we absorb subtle energies through our food, if you read e-mails from your boss whilst eating your lunch, or watch soaps on TV during your evening meal, you will absorb some of that trauma through your food. Your state of mind has a direct effect on the efficiency of your digestion. If you can't enjoy a relaxed environment, cultivate a serene state of mind as you eat. As before, eat with complete awareness. Notice the smells, colours and tastes, chew your food properly and your body will love you for it, rewarding you with efficient, complete digestion and energy.

Who is doing the eating: food and constitution

I've already mentioned that Ayurveda considers food from an energetic point of view based upon taste. It considers six tastes and their effect on each of the doshas. A taste can be aggravating or pacifying in its action on each of the constitutions. Choosing a diet that limits the food substances that aggravate your constitution but includes those that help to pacify and balance will improve your digestion, energy levels and overall health. The following table summarises the effect of each taste on the three doshas.

Taste	Vata	Pitta	Kapha
Sweet	↓	↓	↑
Sour	↓	↑	↑
Salt	↓	↑	↑
Pungent	↑	↑	↓
Bitter	↑	↓	↓
Astringent	↑	↓	↓

↑ Aggravates   ↓ Pacifies

Foods for the three constitutions

Here is a list of foods for constitutions and their effect on each dosha. This will help you to create a balanced diet for your particular type. Ayurveda says that we should have a mix of tastes and colours at each meal ensuring an optimum nutritional balance. We will discuss this in a little more detail in the next section.

I said earlier that most people have a mixed constitution and that it's rare for individuals to be purely of one doshic type. The advice here is a practical simplification of a more complex system, and therefore should be taken as a general guide for those displaying strong constitutional characteristics.

Vata

Generally sweet, sour and salty foods are good. They satisfy the system and reduce insecurity about being well fed. Bitter, pungent and astringent foods are less good as they dry the system and intensify emotional instability. Large amounts of any taste should be avoided as vata is aggravated by excess.

	Pacifying		Aggravating
Fruits	All sweet fruits Apricots Avocado Bananas Berries Cherries Coconut Fresh figs Grapefruit Grapes	Lemons Mango Melon Nectarines Oranges Papaya Peaches Pineapples Plums	All dried fruits Apples Cranberries Pears Pomegranate
Vegetables	All cooked vegetables Asparagus Beets Carrots Garlic Green beans Cooked onion	Sweet potato Radishes Zucchini	All raw vegetables Broccoli Brussels sprouts Cabbage Cauliflower Celery Lettuce Peas
Grains	Cooked oats Rice Wheat (but heavy and can cause allergies)		Barley Buckwheat Corn Millet Dry oats Rye
Animal foods	Beef Chicken Turkey Eggs Seafood		Lamb Pork Rabbit Venison
Legumes	(Cook well with garlic, ginger and turmeric) Red lentils Chickpeas Mung beans Tofu		
Dairy	All dairy ok in moderation		
Seeds and nuts	All seeds and nuts ok in moderation		
Herbs and spices	Asafoetida Ginger Pepper Mustard	Fenugreek Cinnamon Coriander Cumin	
Oils	Sesame Coconut	Mustard	Sunflower
Others	Raw honey All sweeteners except white sugar		Tobacco Sugar Caffeine

Pitta

Generally sweet, bitter and astringent tastes are good. Sour, salty and pungent (the hot tastes) should be avoided, particularly meat, alcohol, eggs and salt. Grains, fruit and vegetables cool the pitta heat and should form the majority of the pitta diet.

	Pacifying		Aggravating
Fruits	All sweet fruits Apples Apricots Avocado Coconut Figs Dark grapes Mango Melon Nectarines Oranges (sweet)	Pears Pineapple (sweet) Plums (sweet) Pomegranate Prunes Raisins	All sour fruits Berries Bananas Cranberries Grapefruit Grapes (green) Lemons Oranges (sour) Papaya Pineapple (sour) Plums (sour)
Vegetables	All sweet and bitter vegetables Asparagus Broccoli Brussels sprouts Cabbage Cucumber Cauliflower	Celery Green beans Leafy greens Lettuce Mushrooms Potatoes Peas Peppers (green)	All pungent vegetables Beets Carrots Aubergine Onions (uncooked) Peppers (hot) Radishes Tomatoes (sour)
Grains	Barley (best – cooling and drying and reduces stomach acid) Oats (cooked) Rice Wheat (avoid yeasted breads – unyeasted are ok)		Buckwheat Corn Millet Oats (dry) Rice (brown) Rye
Animal foods	Chicken Turkey Egg white		Beef Pork Egg yolk Seafood Lamb
Legumes	Black lentils Chick peas	Mung beans Tofu	Red lentils
Dairy	Butter (unsalted) Cottage cheese Ghee Milk		Buttermilk Cheese Sour cream Yogurt
Seeds and nuts	Coconut Sunflower Pumpkin	Sesame (in moderation)	
Herbs and spices	Coriander Cinnamon Cardamom Fennel	Turmeric Clove	Chillies Pepper Mustard Fenugreek
Oils	Coconut Olive Sunflower	Soy Sesame (in moderation)	Almond Corn Safflower
Others			Alcohol Tobacco Coffee

Kapha

Generally bitter, pungent and astringent food that invigorates bodies and minds. Sweet, sour and salty substances should be avoided. Kapha types should never eat fried or greasy foods and should avoid dairy and fat. They should also limit the amount of food they eat.

	Pacifying		Aggravating
Fruits	Apples Apricots Berries Cherries Cranberries Figs (dry) Mango Peaches Pears Pomegranate Prunes Raisins		All sweet and sour fruits Avocado Bananas Coconut Figs (fresh) Grapefruit Grapes Lemons Melon Oranges Papaya Pineapples Plums
Vegetables	All pungent and bitter vegetables Asparagus Beets Broccoli Brussel sprouts Cabbage Carrots Cauliflower Celery Aubergine	Garlic Leafy greens Lettuce Mushrooms Onions Peas Peppers Potatoes Radishes Spinach	All sweet and juicy vegetables Cucumber Potatoes (sweet) Tomatoes
Grains	Barley Corn Millet	Oats (dry) Rice	Oats (cooked) Wheat
Animal foods	Chicken Turkey Shrimp		Beef Seafood Lamb Pork
Legumes	All legumes especially; Black beans	Pinto beans Red lentils	Kidney beans Black lentils Soy beans
Dairy	Ghee Goat's milk		Most dairy is too heavy and cooling
Seeds and nuts	Sunflower Pumpkin (In moderation)		The energy of nuts and seeds can be heavy and oily for kaphas
Herbs and spices	All spices particularly: Ginger, Garlic		Salt
Oils	No oils		(Should generally be avoided but ok in moderation) Almond Corn Sunflower (All in small amounts)
Others	Raw honey		Sweet substances should be avoided

What we eat

I will provide some simple generic rules concerning different types of food that apply to all constitutions. You can then add the details of the foods appropriate for each type to adapt the general principles to your own needs. Ayurvedic recommendations are not described in terms of proteins, carbohydrates and fats as with conventional nutrition, but there are some significant similarities. It's therefore worth expressing the system in a way that's accessible to most people. By ensuring that your eating fits the profile in the Skilful Eating triangle below, you will also ensure you have the appropriate mix of tastes in your diet.

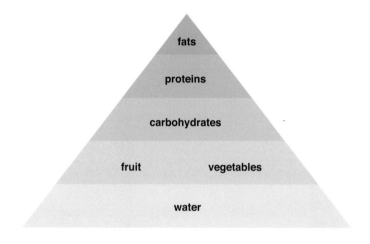

Water

Boosting your intake of water is a simple but powerful purification technique. Most of us do not drink enough water and our sensitivity to thirst can diminish with age. The optimum amount is around 2 litres each day. If you are eating the recommended amount of fruit and vegetables, then you are probably getting about 1 litre of water through your food. This means you need to be drinking at least 1 litre every day, preferably in the form of pure fresh water, through fruit or herb teas, or diluted fruit juice. All constitutions should avoid drinking tea, coffee or alcohol.

Drinking appropriate amounts of water throughout the day will help you to remove toxins, lose unwanted weight, have more energy and look younger. One test as to whether you have the quantity right is that you should feel the need to empty your bladder about every two hours. Drink fresh, pure water but try to avoid very cold water or significant amounts during a meal as it dilutes the gastric juices, dousing the digestive fire.

● Drink at least 1 litre of fresh pure water, herb or fruit tea or diluted fruit juice every day

● Avoid tea, coffee and alcohol.

Fruit and vegetables

As we are talking about energy here, ensure that at least half of your diet contains foods brimming with natural life force. In other words fresh, live food of the kind that can go off if not eaten immediately. In Ayurvedic terms, any processing alters the taste and quality of the food, changing its energetic effects. A good rule is to eat food as close to its natural form as possible. The only exception is for strong vata types who tend to digest vegetables better with some light cooking, preferably steaming.

● Eat at least five portions of fruit and vegetables every day – see the list for those best for your constitution

● Include as much live food as possible in your diet daily – as close to its natural form as possible

● Eat plenty of vegetables that contain the seed, as they are usually packed with nutrients for growing the next generation – examples include peas and beans.

Carbohydrates

Ayurveda suggests that there should be a predominance of sweet taste in your diet. This should not be interpreted as the sweetness associated with refined sugar, but substances that in modern terms could be classified as complex carbohydrates. This would include many of the fruit and vegetables as well as food such as rice and wheat.

● This food group should make up about 70% of your total dietary intake

● Wholegrains, particularly rice, are considered to be pure (*satvic*) in Ayurveda and at least 3 portions a day should be included in your diet.

Proteins

Although Ayurveda does not prohibit the use of meat in the diet, it does recommend that a *satvic* (pure) diet be consumed for optimum physical and mental health. A *satvic* diet is light and easy to digest, usually vegetarian and facilitates the efficient production of ojas and clarity of mental processes. The amount of animal protein should be limited to about three portions each week and most protein sources should be sought through beans and lentils.

● Eat vegetable-based proteins, beans, lentils, tofu, quinoa

● Animal proteins tend to be high in saturated fats so limit consumption to three times per week and eat during the lunchtime meal.

Fats

Ayurveda does suggest a meal be unctuous or moist, and recommends a small amount of pure oil of ghee (clarified butter). Although the high (saturated) fat content is an area for concern in modern terms, it acknowledges that certain fats are essential for proper functioning. Essential fats are best acquired from seeds and nuts or pure cold-pressed oils.

● Eat at least 1 heaped tablespoon of seeds or nuts each day

● Eat at least 1 tablespoon of pure cold-pressed seed oil each day (can be sunflower, sesame, etc)

● If cooking with oils, do not heat them too much and use pure ghee if possible.

Skilful Eating – Summary of Key Skills

Understand your emotional relationship with food
- Understand your food history
- Eat for health, energy and joy, not comfort or compensation

Listen to your body
- Finish your meals feeling light but satisfied
- Eat like a child – only as much as your body needs and only when you are hungry
- Observe and respond to your digestive indicators
- Get to know your constitution and include food groups that pacify your predominant dosha
- Eat with complete awareness

Follow the skilful energy cycle
- Eat a light but substantial breakfast full of fresh fruit, mixed seeds and wholegrains
- Make lunch the main meal of the day – if you are going to eat animal proteins, take them during this meal
- The evening meal should be light, vegetarian and early, and no later than 20.00
- Put the ceremony back into your eating habits
- Avoid eating at your desk or watching television

Skilful use of food
- Apply diversity to your diet – balance nutrients, colours and include all six tastes
- Drink at least 1 litre of water, herbal or fruit tea each day
- Avoid excess caffeine as it causes tension in the body and hyperactivity in the mind – drinking coffee when under stress worsens the situation so drink it in moderation!
- Avoid excess alcohol as it creates an acidic imbalance in the stomach and also dulls the senses
- Eat at least 5 portions of fresh fruit and vegetables every day
- Eat as much live food as possible and include lots of seed vegetables
- Eat at least 3 servings of complex carbohydrate each day
- Minimise refined sugars as it can suppress the digestive process and cause hyperactivity, creating imbalance in the body and mind – this is particularly important at night as it may cause insomnia.
- Eat 3 servings of protein, such as lentils or beans each day and avoid excess animal source proteins
- Eat at least 1 tablespoon of pure cold-pressed seed oil, or ground seeds, or nuts every day
- Include herbs and spices according to your constitution; include garlic, ginger, cumin, coriander, turmeric, etc – this will help to include all six tastes
- Make eating a joyful experience!

skilful activity

Rhythms in nature

We have already introduced the concept of daily energy cycles in Skilful Eating. Here we are still concerned with providing you with optimum levels of energy and will discuss in a little more detail how to use the cycles described in Ayurveda.

There are certain rhythms in nature that are reflected in daily, seasonal and time-of-life cycles. Ayurveda describes these cycles that our physiology undergoes. With a little knowledge and application it is possible to utilise the fluctuation of these energies to enhance our health. For example, we have already described how our digestive fire peaks for a few hours during the day. By aligning our main meal with this period, we can maximise the efficiency of our digestion. Also, certain doshas become dominant throughout our lives, depending upon our age and state of health. Kapha dosha predominates in childhood, from birth to about 25 when the main physical growth and development occurs. Pitta is dominant from 25 to about 60 and vata takes over in old age, as our body tissues tend to weaken and lose some of their elasticity. These periods are approximate but Charaka, one of the authors of an important Ayurvedic text, states that the average life span of a human should be between 100 and 120 years, with good health and vigour for most of this period. Because few of us ever achieve this does not mean that we should not set our expectations high!

Daily cycles

Let's have another look at each of the daily cycles and describe some other things we can do during each period.

Kapha period: 06.00 – 10.00

● Remember that this period can be heavy and sluggish due to the predominance of kapha. To bring lightness and energy to this period consider the following routine:

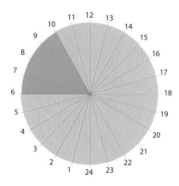

The wake-up routine

● **Rising during vata period:** Yogis state that the healthiest time of the day to rise is during *Brahma Muhurta* – or just before sunrise! By rising before 6.00am you may find you are more alert and awake than when getting up during the kapha period. Try it and see if it makes a difference!

● **Challenge your comfort zone:** Splash your face seven times with cool water. This disperses residual pitta energy. Seven is an auspicious number in yoga, as it relates to the energy centres in the body. It is also good to start the day by challenging yourself to get out of your comfort zone. Starting the day in this way will help you to carry that attitude into the day.

● **The 15-minute routine:** This is the best time of day to complete your sequence of postures, breathing and visualisation exercises described below. All of these activities counteract kapha and bring lightness to the body and calmness to the mind.

● **Elimination:** Kapha is pacified by cleansing the body and getting rid of waste products. If you have followed the Skilful Eating suggestions and completed your 15-minute routine, I'm sure that your body will be ready to eliminate its waste during this period. If you do rise before 6.00am, elimination will most likely occur then, as vata is responsible for the natural urges.

● **Cleansing routine:** Showering is a natural cleansing process and the flow of warm water on your skin will also pacify the cold characteristic of kapha.

● **Oil application:** Following your shower or bath consider rubbing a small amount of oil into your skin. Self massage, particularly around the joints, will stimulate blood and energy flow. Use oil that is appropriate for your constitution: sesame for vatas, sandalwood for pittas and mustard for kaphas. Rub a little into your ears as there are some important energy channels here and this simple oil massage will protect the whole body and stimulate all of your senses.

● Finish your routine by rubbing a small amount of the oil inside your nostrils. Ayurveda considers the nose as the pathway to the brain and this will ensure mental clarity as well as cleaning the sinuses.

● **Scrape your tongue:** That layer of fuzz on your tongue is ama, and you should avoid ingesting it with your food. Tongue scraping should be done from back to front and not only gets rid of ama, but also stimulates the taste buds and awakens your senses.

● After eating a light breakfast, you are ready to head into work with a lightness and energy that will set the tone for the rest of your day.

● **Influence your thoughts:** Write your personal goals and affirmations before you are influenced by anything else (See Skilful Thinking).

The daily yoga routine

Your body was designed for movement. Exercise places the body under beneficial stress, improving physical and mental vitality and performance. For optimum health and performance, you need exercise – it is as simple as that!

Yoga postures are not strictly exercises. They are techniques that place the body in positions that increase awareness, relaxation and concentration as well as developing good health by stretching, massaging and stimulating the physical and energetic body. If done with awareness and control, the following suggested routines will take no more than 10 minutes to complete. The first routine is very gentle, the second slightly more dynamic.

As with any exercise programme, you need to consult your doctor before undertaking either routine. This is particularly important if you have suffered from any back, neck or heart problems, or if you are pregnant. The author, publisher and distributors of this book disclaim any liability or loss in connection with the exercises or material contained within.

Gentle yoga routine

Starting position (calibrate awareness and focus)

Preparation
● Lie on your back.

● Bring your awareness to your breath, your inhalation and exhalation.

● Follow 6 breaths counting down from 6 to 1.

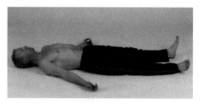

Tips
● Centre your senses and awareness on your practice and try not to be distracted by anything else.

● Keep this sense of awareness through the practice and beyond.

Arms overhead stretch (a stretch for your shoulders, chest and back)

Preparation

● Lie on your back with legs bent, feet on the floor and arms beside you.

Practice

● Inhaling, raise your arms up overhead behind.

● Hold the breath for a second. Allow your arms to be fully supported by the floor so that your neck and shoulder muscles can relax.

● Exhaling, lower your arms back down to the sides of your body.

Repeat 3 times

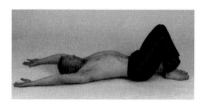

Tips

● Maintain the length in your neck by keeping your chin gently tucked in.

● Maintain the curve in your lower back and the neutral position of your pelvis by gently contracting your deep abdominal muscles.

● If your arms don't touch the floor behind you then bend your elbows to release your neck and shoulders.

Spinal rock (a gentle massage for the muscles of your back)

Preparation

● Lie on your back with legs bent, feet on the floor and arms beside you.

Practice

● Draw your thighs in towards your abdomen.

● Rest your hands over your knees and gently rock from side to side.

Practise for 1 minute

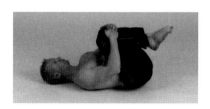

Tips

● The closer you draw your thighs in towards your abdomen the further up your back you will feel the effects of the massage.

Knee hug (stretch for buttocks and lower back)

Preparation

● Lie on your back with legs bent, feet on the floor and arms beside you.

● Draw your thighs in towards your abdomen.

● Gently rest your right hand on your right knee and left hand on your left knee.

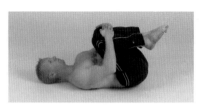

Repeat 3 times

Practice

● Exhaling, bend your arms and allow your thighs to be drawn towards your chest and abdomen.

● Inhaling, straighten your arms and allow your thighs to move away from your chest and abdomen.

Tips

● Maintain the length in your neck by keeping your chin gently tucked in.

● Keep your shoulders and hands relaxed.

Spinal twist (stretch for the ribs and deep muscles of the back)

Preparation

● Lie on your back with legs bent, feet on the floor and arms at right angles to your body with the palms turned down.

Practice

● Exhaling, lower your knees to the left as you rotate your head to the right.

● Stay for 1 breath.

● Inhaling, bring your knees back to the centre and your head facing forward.

● Exhaling, lower your knees to the right and rotate your head to the left.

● Stay for one breath.

● Inhaling, bring your knees back to the centre and turn your head to face forward.

● Exhaling, lower your arms back down to the sides of your body.

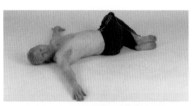

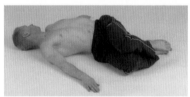

Repeat 2 times to each side

Tips

● Ensure you rest your legs and arms while in the posture. Try to release any unnecessary tension.

● As you breathe whilst in the posture, feel rib cage expand and contract.

Straight leg raise (stretch for backs of the legs)

Preparation

● Lie on your back with legs bent, feet on the floor and arms beside you.

● Draw your right thigh in towards your abdomen and rest your hands around the back of the right knee.

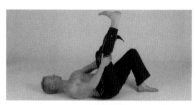

Practice

● Breathe in. Straighten your leg, pushing through the heel of your foot and drawing your toes in towards you. Feel the stretch up the back of your leg and behind your ankle.

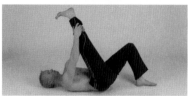

● Exhaling, draw your thigh back in towards your abdomen and hug.

Repeat 3 times each side

Tips

● Maintain the length in your neck by keeping your chin gently tucked in.

● Maintain the curve in your lower back and the neutral position of your pelvis by gently contracting your deep abdominal muscles.

Two foot support or bridge (stretch the front of the body and mobilise the spine)

Preparation

● Lie on your back with legs bent, feet on the floor and arms beside you.

Practice

● Inhaling, lift your pelvis, your lower back, your middle back, and then upper back off the floor. **Stop if there is any discomfort in the neck or lower back.**

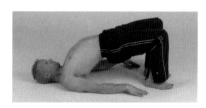

Repeat 3 times

● Exhaling, lower your upper back, then middle back, and then lower back and pelvis back down onto the floor.

Tips

● Gently push your shoulders down into the floor as you lift your back.

● Try to 'peel' your spine off the floor vertebra by vertebra.

Crunches (strengthens abdominal muscles)

Preparation

● Lie on your back with legs bent, feet on the floor and arms overhead behind you, resting on the floor.

Practice

● Exhaling, first raise your arms off the floor to either side of your knees. When necessary lift the back of your head off the floor and finally shoulders.

● Inhaling, first lower your shoulders, then the back of your head and then arms back overhead behind you.

Repeat 4 times

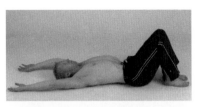
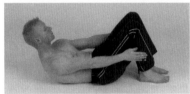

Tips

● Maintain the curve in your lower back and the neutral position of your pelvis by gently contracting your deep abdominal muscles throughout the movement.

Backward bend (stretch for the front of the body and spine)

Preparation

● Lie on your front with your hands level with your shoulders, forearms resting on the floor and forehead resting on the floor.

● Gently rock from side to side to relax your buttocks and muscles of your back.

Practice

● Inhaling. Lift head and chest off the floor and rest supported by your forearms with your back muscles totally relaxed.

● Stay for 2 – 3 breaths.

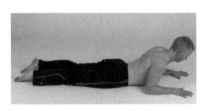

● Exhaling. Slowly lower your chest and head back down to the floor.

Repeat 2 times

Tips

● Gently rock from side to side in the posture if necessary to keep back muscles relaxed.

Downward dog pose (good 'all rounder' – strengthens and stretches the body)

Preparation

● Sit on your heels with forehead and forearms resting on the floor.

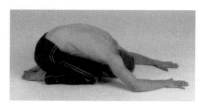

Practice

● Inhaling, come up on to the hands and knees, knees under the hips, hands under the shoulders. Keep the spine long.

● Exhaling, lift pelvis off the floor, upwards and backwards and straighten legs and arms.

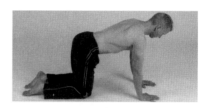

● Inhaling, lower yourself back down onto your hands and knees.

● Exhaling, sit back down onto your heels, forehead and forearms resting on the floor.

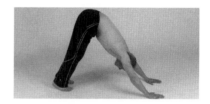

Repeat 3 – 6 times

Tips

● Keep feet shoulder width apart.

● Focus on relaxing and lengthening the area between your shoulder blades while in the posture.

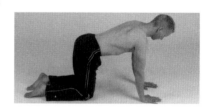

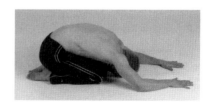

Relaxation posture (allow your body to absorb the benefits of the practice)

● Lie on your back.

● Bring your awareness to your breath, your inhalation and exhalation.

● Follow 12 breaths counting down from 12 to 1.

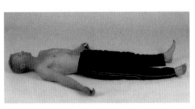

Tips

● Place a cushion under your knees if your lower back feels tense.

● Place a thin pillow under your head if your neck feels compressed.

Complete the practice by completing the breathing and visualisation exercises described on pages 78 and 79.

Dynamic yoga routine

Centring position

● Lie on your back.

● Bring your awareness to your breath, your inhalation and exhalation.

● Follow 6 breaths counting down from 6 to 1.

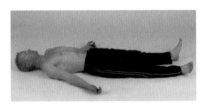

Tips

● Centre your senses and awareness on your practice and try not to be distracted by anything else.

● Keep this sense of awareness through the practice and beyond.

Starting position

● Stand tall with feet together, muscles above the knees lifting, hips tilted forwards and shoulder blades rolled down the back.

● There is a feeling of openness and balance in this posture.

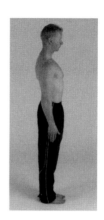

Position 1

● Inhale as the arms rise above the head and the palms come together.

● Turn the gaze up towards the thumbs to open the throat area.

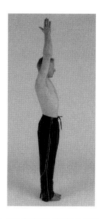

Position 2

● Hold the breath as the arms drop behind the head.

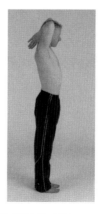

Position 3

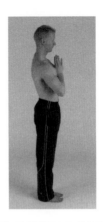

● Still holding the breath, bring the hands into 'prayer position' on the chest.

Position 4

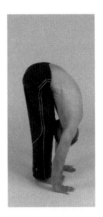

● Exhale and bend forwards.

● Keep the spine long and relaxed.

● Bring the hands to a point on the legs where they feel comfortable, or if they reach the floor put the palms flat either side of the feet.

Position 5

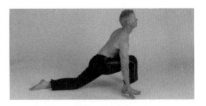

● Inhale as the left foot reaches back as far as possible.

● The left knee is in contact with the floor; the right knee is over the right heel to protect the knee joint.

● Turn the gaze upwards to open the throat and the heart area.

Position 6

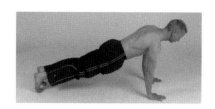

- Step back with the right foot.

- There should be about six inches between feet and a straight line throughout the body.

- Hold the breath in this position.

Position 7

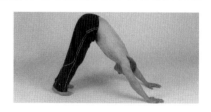

- Exhale as the hips push up and back into 'downward dog' position.

- Push the heels down to the floor; keep the legs straight if you can.

- Push the chest down towards the feet – this lengthens and flattens the back.

- The arms are straight and the palms pushed into the floor with the fingers spread.

- Keep the abdomen pulled in slightly and the chin tucked into the chest.

- Hold this position for at least two full breaths.

Position 8

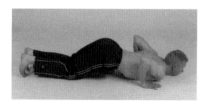

- On exhaling, drop the body into a position where the hands, feet, knees, chest and chin are in contact with the floor.

- Pause very briefly.

Position 9

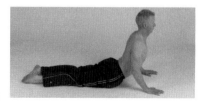

- Inhale. Slide the body forward and upward opening the chest and the throat.

- The legs and hips remain in contact with the floor.

- The weight pushes into the palms and the shoulders roll down the back opening up the heart area.

Position 10

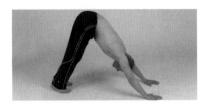

● Exhale and push the hips backward and upwards into the downward dog position once more.

● There is no 'hold' this time.

Position 11

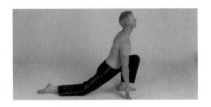

● Inhale, bringing the left foot forward to a position between the hands.

● Lift the gaze to open the throat and the heart areas.

Position 12

● Exhaling, bring the right foot forward next to the left and into the forward bend position once more.

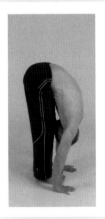

Position 13

● Inhale, straightening the body and bringing the arms over the head with palms together.

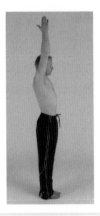

Position 14

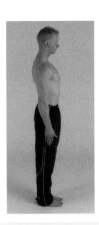

● Exhale, lowering the arms to the side of the body ready for the next round.

General tips

● This is a dynamic sequence where the breath drives the movement. Try and develop a flowing rhythm for the whole sequence.

● The above sequence is for the left side; balance the body by repeating the sequence on the right side.

● Do three sequences either side, making six rounds in all.

● Focus on the breath rather than the postures. Precision in the postures will come with time and practice.

Position 15

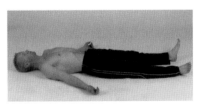

● Lie on your back.

● Bring your awareness to your breath, your inhalation and exhalation.

● Follow 12 breaths counting down from 12 to 1.

Tips

● Place a cushion under your knees if your lower back feels tense.

● Place a thin pillow under your head if your neck feels compressed.

Complete the practice by completing the breathing and visualisation exercises described on pages 78 and 79.

Pitta period 10.00 – 14.00

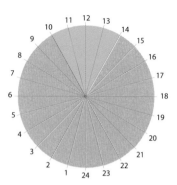

During this active pitta period all digestive processes, both physical and mental, will be high.

- A good period for intellectual activities, particularly the morning period, as there will be a feeling of lightness and energy. The best work of the day can often be done here.

- Meeting with pitta types just before lunch can sometimes be counterproductive – if they are hungry they can be irritable and fiery. Arrange a working lunch instead!

- Ideally, the main meal of the day should be eaten during this period. It should follow the good practice guidelines given in the Skilful Eating section.

- No sluggishness should be felt after lunch if the correct food has been consumed. Daytime sleep should be avoided as it increases kapha and reduces agni.

Working with Awareness

I've already mentioned that your body was designed to move. We often suffer more in the workplace than anywhere else, as this is the place we get stressed and sit for long periods, often in positions that are harmful. Sitting in an office in front of a computer prevents your body and mind from doing what they're designed to do and performing at their best. Simple movement will help your digestive processes and improve your energy levels during periods of the day when they feel low. Being in touch with your body means that you should be aware of your physical and energetic needs at all times.

Aim to be aware of your posture as you sit, and of any points of stress or tension in your body. You should move at least every half hour just for a few minutes; programme a screen saver or put a post-it note on your desk to remind you.

After eating, Ayurveda says that you should take at least a hundred steps to aid your digestive process. If you cannot walk around, complete some of the simple desktop yoga exercises that follow.

Movement improves our digestion by increasing agni; it helps to improve circulation, eliminate waste products and balance all three doshas. It is easy if we are sat at a desk to complete these simple but powerful exercises, starting at your neck and moving down your body to your legs, moving all major muscle groups and joints.

Desktop yoga

All stretches should feel enjoyable and comfortable.
Always stop if in any discomfort.

Neck

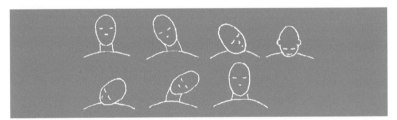

Neck rolls
- Drop your shoulders down.
- Fix shoulders and take your ear to shoulder.
- Roll chin to chest and take ear to other shoulder.
- Repeat moving in the other direction.
- Avoid dropping head backwards.

Shoulders

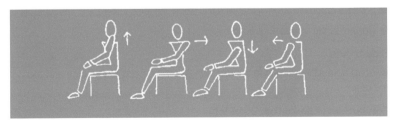

Shoulder rolls
- Roll shoulders up towards your ears.
- Roll shoulders back/squeeze shoulder blades.

- Roll shoulders downwards.
- Roll shoulders forwards.
- Repeat 3 times backwards. Repeat 3 times forwards.

Shoulder shrugs

- Lift shoulders to ears. Squeeze tight.
- Exhale, drop and relax. Repeat 3 times.

Back

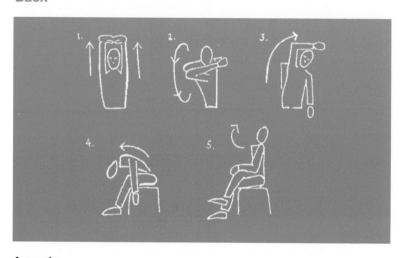

Arm raise

- Interlace fingers and turn hands palm outwards.
- Lift arms above head. Hold 3 breaths.
- Exhaling, release arms to the sides of the body. Repeat 3 times.

Elbow circles (upper back stretch)

- Clasp back of the neck, elbows pointing forwards.
- Scribe a gradually larger spiral with the elbow, keeping lower back and hips still.
- Repeat in the opposite direction.

Side bends

- Keep both sitting bones in contact with the chair; bend to one side and then the other.

Forward bend (lower back stretch)

- Sit on a chair, relax the body forwards and rest the chest and abdomen on thighs.

Spinal twist

● Lengthen and straighten spine.

● Cross right leg over left and rotate right.

● Cross left leg over right and rotate left.

Hands and wrists

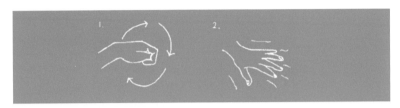

Wrist rotations

● Bend thumbs into palms of hands and close fingers over them. Rotate fists in one direction and then the other.

Hand and wrist shakes

● Open your fingers and shake hands and wrists.

Legs

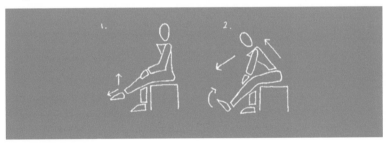

Calf stretch and pump

● Straighten one leg out in front.

● Point toes away and stretch front of leg.

● Pull back the toes, push into heel and stretch calf.

Hamstring stretch

● Straighten out one leg.

● Tilt pelvis forwards.

● Lean forwards with chin tucked and spine straight.

● Repeat other side.

Vata period 14.00 – 18.00

If appropriate food has been eaten, the early part of digestion should be well underway and you should be feeling light.

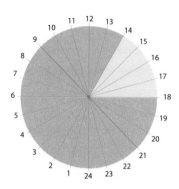

● Again, a good period for activity due to the dynamic nature of vata.

● Vata is cold and dry in nature so this can be countered by consuming hot drinks. Stimulants such as tea or coffee should be avoided if possible. Try hot ginger tea or something similar – or see the list in the Skilful Eating section.

● Vata periods can give rise to anxiety due to the fluctuating nature of the energy force. If you feel this, then do the short breathing exercises or the visualisation described below.

Breathing and Visualisation

Yoga not only includes physical movement, but active use of the breath and positive control of our mental processes. Following the desktop yoga, try the following simple breathing techniques:

● **Yogic breath:** Most of us do not utilise our full breathing capacity, particularly when we are stressed. A full inhalation should engage your diaphragm and push out your abdomen; your ribs should expand outwards and backwards and your chest rise towards your neck. Exhalation should reverse this process. Practise getting this gentle wave-like movement without straining. Once you have the movement flowing and natural, inhale for a count of five, hold for a count of five and breathe out for a count of ten. Take about five of these breaths and do this whenever you are feeling stressed or anxious.

● **Alternate nostril breathing:** This is a technique that may take a little more practice, but once mastered helps to combat stress, clear the sinuses, raise your body temperature and balance the body's three energy forces. Place your index finger of your right hand between your eyebrows, your thumb on your right nostril and your ring finger on your left nostril. Closing your right nostril, breathe in your left for a count of five (using your full yogic breath as described above). Close your left nostril and breathe out of your right for a count of ten. Breathe in through the right nostril for a count of five and then out left for a count of ten. This is one round. Complete three rounds.

● **Energetic light visualisation:** Find a few quiet moments each day to use visualisation to bring you positive energy. Sit in a quiet place and take a deep breath. Take your mind to your eyelids and, on exhaling, feel the tension drain from your body: from your eyelids, over your head, down your body and out through your feet. Take another deep breath and, on exhaling, relax your mind as you see yourself slide into a personal sanctuary such as a beautiful garden. Visualise yourself sat there and bring a healing light into your body. See it fill you from the top of your head to the tips of your toes, until it radiates from your skin. Keep this glowing energy with you throughout the day and top it up often.

Kapha period 18.00 – 22.00

This second kapha period of the day means that often lethargy can set in. Again, daytime sleep should be avoided as it may affect night sleep and cause an imbalance of kapha dosha.

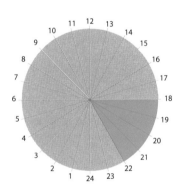

● Eat a light evening meal when the afternoon meal has been digested, following the guidelines provided in Skilful Eating.

● Another good period for exercise as physical activity counters the heavy kapha energy.

The 15-Minute Routine   The 15-minute routine consists of:

● 10 Minutes of yoga postures – either the gentle routine on page 62 or the dynamic routine on page 68

● 3 Minutes of breathing exercises – either the yogic breath or the alternate nostril breathing

● 2 Minutes of energetic light visualisations

This simple, but highly effective routine should be completed once each day, ideally during one of the kapha periods and preferably first thing in the morning. Follow this routine for 30 days and I guarantee you will notice a difference in your energy and outlook.

Using constitution in the workplace

Skilful activity is not only about the smart utilisation of energy cycles; it is also about understanding and utilising our natural abilities to the full. Our vocation is influenced by our values, beliefs and desires for the future, all of which we will explore in detail in the next section. It is also driven by inherent characteristics. These are influenced by our personal mind/body type – our constitution.

Earlier we looked at some of the general characteristics of each personality type. Let's now look specifically at how this is relevant to our relationships, particularly those in the workplace. If we know about a person's basic values – the things that motivate them, the things that create stress and the areas where they have inherent skills – then we can use this information to positively influence our relationship with them. The differences between the types may manifest themselves in many ways: the areas that individuals like to focus their attention on, the way that they take in information, the environment they like to work in, the type of work they like and the lifestyle they prefer to adopt. This information can help us be a little more skilful about allocating tasks to team members or drive the way we communicate to different individuals. For example, we may be a little more prescriptive in requesting progress feedback from a vata type who, left to their own devices, may not be particularly proactive in their communication. With a kapha type however, they may need more detail in the beginning to get started, but will probably give frequent written communication without being asked.

For our purposes, one of the important uses of this information is knowing what types of work and which environments are likely to produce a stressful response from different individuals. Sometimes, simply understanding these basic motivating factors can give us greater tolerance or patience towards an individual, even if their style does not match our own. Simply put, if there is a misalignment between people's basic needs and the environment they are working in then stress results. Understanding these things in advance can allow us to avoid or manage such results. Conversely, when we get consistency between values and activity then amazing results are possible.

Similar principles are also applicable to teams. For particular projects, it is possible to design the profile of the team members to give the most beneficial outcome. For example, you will get a very high-energy team if you fill it with vata types, but you may find that very little planning gets done and they may head off in different directions. This can be balanced by adding a kapha type who will insist on more planning and communication.

A team made exclusively of kaphas however, may plan and think about the process, but never actually get round to doing anything. So the balance in teams is important and, if managed skilfully, can give excellent results.

Let's have a look at the particular attributes of each type and how they relate to the working environment in terms of the things they can contribute, their leadership styles and any potential limitations that may need to be strengthened.

Vata in the Workplace

Contribution to an organisation

- Fast tracks projects
- Action-orientated, capable of rapid results
- Goal-orientated
- Quick thinking and imaginative with good problem solving skills

Leadership style

- Can be inspiring, energetic and enthusiastic
- Usually finds good reasons for whatever he/she wants
- Improvises rather than plans
- Can sometimes lack regular communication or feedback to team members

Preferred work environment

- Likes variety and action
- May prefer to communicate by talking rather than writing
- Enthusiastic, but tends to work in bursts of energy
- Wants only the essentials to begin his/her work

Potential limitations

- Often lacks concentration, stamina and patience with long slow projects
- Can act impulsively and leap to conclusions
- Has low tolerance for repetitive activities
- Dislikes taking time for precision
- May start too many projects
- Can create confusion through lack of planning

Pitta in the Workplace

Contribution to an organisation

- Strong creativity and idea generation
- Complex problem solving through analysis and critical thinking
- Sharp memory and intellect
- Purposeful beyond pay cheque – living in congruence with values
- Intense and ambitious
- Cuts directly to core issues
- Short and long term intellectual insight

Leadership style

- Tends to be firm and tough minded
- Able to reprimand or fire people when necessary
- Leads through conceptual analysis of problems and goals
- Focused, aware and goal-orientated
- Seeks to interact at an intellectual rather than an emotional level
- Fosters independence in others

Preferred work environment

- Enjoys learning new skills
- Needs to be treated fairly
- Wants to know all about a new job
- Prefers feedback on results and performance
- Flexible until inner values violated
- Doesn't like structures and rules

Potential limitations

- Can overcomplicate or over intellectualise a task
- Can be aggressive, intolerant and confrontational
- Can focus on minor inconsistencies at the expense of teamwork and harmony
- Can turn critical and analytical thinking on people and act impersonally

Kapha in the Workplace

Contribution to an organisation

● Succeeds by perseverance, originality; desires to do whatever is needed

● Excellent memory and stability

● Thorough and precise with good attention to detail

● Loyal, considerate and perceptive lending stability to any group

● Process-orientated

Leadership style

● Respected for firm principles and likely to be honoured and followed for his/her clear convictions

● Quietly forceful, conscientious and concerned with how others feel

● Stable, strong and trustworthy

Preferred work environment

● Likes quiet and concentration

● Can work on one project for a long time without interruption

● May prefer communication to be in writing

● Works best when can plan and follow work

● Likes to work with real rather than abstract issues

Potential limitations

● Sometimes slow to act

● May dislike to interrupt the project he/she is on for a more urgent one

● Doesn't respond well to need for rapid results and may miss deadlines if under short-term pressure

● Can procrastinate and can lack results orientation

Skilful Activity – A Summary of the Key Skills

● Know your constitution and how the daily energy cycles influence you.

● Do the 15-minute routine in the morning – get up a little earlier if necessary, it will be worth it!

● Follow the morning routine and enter the working day feeling positive and vital.

● Get outside your comfort zone consciously at least once per day.

● Understand how your constitution influences your livelihood. Strive for consistency in your activity and basic desires.

● Top up your energy and actively manage your health throughout the day with constant awareness, desktop yoga, breath control and visualisation. See yourself as energetic and healthy and you will be!

three

skilful thinking

EVERYTHING WE HAVE DONE UP UNTIL THIS POINT has been preparation for the work we are about to undertake, the active control of our thinking processes. Real creation takes place when you are in full conscious control of your mind and your body. Everything in your life is created through a set of principles that, once understood and applied, will change the way you view your life experiences. All successful people use these principles, either consciously or unconsciously, to bring about the things they want to achieve. These principles define the cause-and-effect relationships that, once mastered, will help to make you happier, healthier and more successful. You will have a greater sense of power and purpose in your life as you will feel in control of everything you do and the things you wish to achieve. You will grow to understand yourself better and as a result your relationships will improve, including your relationship with yourself!

This section is about bringing these principles to conscious awareness so that you bring the things that you may currently think of as being outside of your control, firmly within your grasp.

The Thinking Triangle

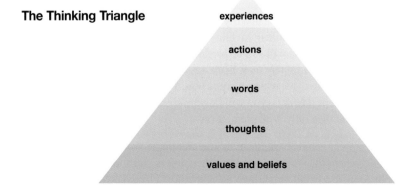

experiences

actions

words

thoughts

values and beliefs

Whether you know it or not, your life is the result of the relationships represented in this triangle. The top level of the triangle represents the things you experience today. These are the results of past and present interactions between the things represented by the lower levels of the triangle.

The things you value and the beliefs that you hold about yourself, others and life in general, drive your thought processes. These thoughts will be expressed in the way you communicate and interact with the world around you, and how you act internally. The things you experience in your life right now are a result of this integrated creative process. This is going on in every moment of every day.

For example, if you hold a *belief* that you usually fail at the things you attempt, then this will be reflected in your *thought* processes about yourself, the *words* you use to communicate with other people and the *actions* you undertake to make things happen or overcome challenges. This belief may lead you to give up before you even try and the things you *experience* in life will flow directly from this belief system. It is this cause-and-effect principle that is at the heart of the whole system.

There is nothing random about the skilful thinking triangle: it works all of the time, not some of the time. It works for everybody, not only the good and the righteous. It does not work for the lucky and bypass the unlucky. It is a natural law, as neutral in its universality as the law of gravity. The only potential limitations are our own understandings, which can constrain our attempts to work constructively with these laws.

The key to designing your life is therefore to actively understand and control the levels in the thinking triangle. Once you have complete congruence between the levels then magical, powerful things will happen.

Most people tackle any process of change from the top, the level of experiences and actions, without giving much thought to what lies beneath. However, if there is inconsistency between the experiences you desire (the top of the triangle) and the underlying belief system (the lower levels of the triangle), you are destined to fail. Your underlying beliefs, values and unconscious thoughts will still be producing the kinds of experience you've always had. Your life may look like a series of random events but in fact it is this system that is working against you. With aims that are inconsistent with your deepest beliefs, you will only be able to change for a short period of time, and then only with great effort.

For example, imagine you want to lose weight. If you wish to achieve this through changing your eating habits, then unless you alter your relationship with food at a belief level, then no permanent changes will be made. You will find yourself dieting for a while in great discomfort as you fight against your most fundamental impulses, but not make any lasting changes to your actions or to your long-term weight loss. For permanent changes to take place, then all levels of the triangle should be congruent. Your belief about your own ability to change, what food means to you and the things you deserve in life need to be altered. Once this new perspective is in place at the base of the triangle, then your behaviour will start to change and you will experience the results you desire.

There is another way of describing the layers of the thinking triangle:

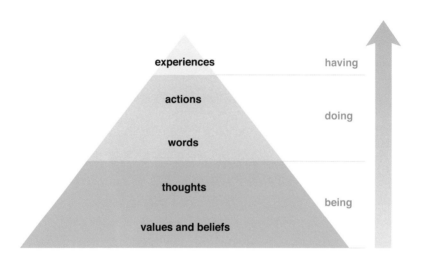

There is a continuum of *being*, *doing* and *having* that describes the same layers of the triangle in a slightly different way. This is important as it is not so much what we are *doing* in our lives that determines what we *have* as what we are *being*! Your state of being is a reflection of your fundamental beliefs and values at this moment. How you are now being determines the life experiences you are having. You are always doing something to satisfy a fundamental value or belief or, in other words, a state of being. This sometimes occurs without you thinking about it. These are automatic responses that reflect a state of being that has already been established. For example when you laugh, cry or become angry you don't think about this response, it is usually spontaneous.

Your body may also undertake action to create a state of being. For example, we *do* the thing called exercise because we wish to *be* fit. This may be driven by a value called the desire to be healthy. We sleep because we want to *be* in the state called rested. We eat to be nourished, and so on. You may go to work to be successful, which satisfies a value called ambition. Someone else may do the same work to be wealthy which satisfies a value called the need for financial security.

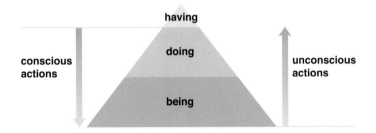

Our body is always doing something, either consciously or unconsciously, that reflects a state of being.

> Go back to the part of the introduction to this book where you defined the area of your life you would most like to improve. If this is not a statement of being, then turn it into one.
>
> For example, if you want greater success or more wealth, then your desired state may be one of *abundance*. If you wanted to lose weight or increase your energy, then your desired state may be *healthy*. If you want better relationships then it may be your state is *loving*. It may be *happy*, *peaceful* or *enlightened* – just ensure that your statement is one of being, rather than doing.
>
> Now, when you have defined it, try to come from that state in every moment, regardless of whatever you're doing.

We have a choice about the state of being that we are in at any moment. The first step therefore in creating a life of your own design is to decide on the state you wish to be in.

Only by creating our life from a state of being will we be expressing who we really are, our most authentic nature. I said earlier that most people attempt to change their lives from the top of the triangle down, by concentrating on doing things or having things that they hope will bring them a desired state of being, such as happiness, wealth, peace, etc. The fact is that you cannot *do* happiness, you can only *be* happy. Similarly, you don't *do* health, you *are* healthy.

I believe that each of us can choose the purpose of our life and create our personal destiny. This is different for each of us. It is our job to uncover and express it as fully as possible. Once achieved, it may appear simply as a sense of connectedness, the feeling of being in harmony with the world around you, of naturally flowing with the actions you undertake. Most of us have met people who feel as though they are doing what they were born to do. This is because they are responding from their true state of being.

Often, such people say that their occupation doesn't feel like work – they feel they're being paid for what they love to do! They are passionate about their lives because what they are is in harmony with what they do. In fact, when the spiritual writer Neale Donald Walsh writes that 'passion is the love of turning being into action', he is saying that this harmony is passion.

Through the process of aligning all of the layers of the thinking triangle, you will be purposefully creating your life experiences from a chosen state of being.

The following principles are about getting in touch with your current state of being at the level of your beliefs and values, and deciding whether this state gives you the experiences you want. If not, this section of the book will provide some tools and techniques to make positive changes.

The seven principles of being

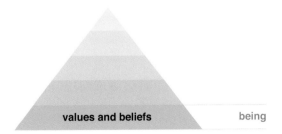

being

1 Know your values

Your life values are those things that are of fundamental importance to you. They provide you with a sense of right or wrong that offers a basic foundation for making decisions. Many people are not clear about their values and therefore often end up making poor decisions about things that are important, such as their career or relationships. They then wonder why things never seem to work out for them. Determining what your current values are is a crucial part of the creative process. This will allow you to recognise the things that are driving your life experiences and to assess whether they serve you in a way consistent with the future you wish to create.

Have a look at the following list and decide your top three values and put them in priority order.

Achievement	Involvement
Adventure	Love
Affection	Loyalty
Comfort	Passion
Competitiveness	Personal development
Cooperation	Pleasure
Creativity	Power
Fame	Recognition
Family happiness	Responsibility
Freedom	Security
Friendship	Self respect
Harmony	Spirituality
Health	Success
Integrity	Wealth
Intimacy	Wisdom

I am sure you looked at the list and identified many that were important to you. However, we all have a hierarchy of values where some are more important than others. If you are to identify your state of being you must recognise that there is often a difference between your conscious thoughts and your deeper values. We get a more accurate picture of our state of being by looking at our *actions*. One of the functions of your conscious thinking mind is to project an image of yourself to the outside world; to produce a personal identity that will maintain a level of protection against potential threat. For this reason, you may attempt to project an image that does not necessarily match with your true self. This may reflect a value that you would *like* to have, or feel that you *should* have, rather than one that is truly yours. However, your body will usually respond unconsciously to the cues from your sub-conscious mind in the form of emotions or action. It is your behaviour that expresses your values.

For example, many people on my workshops tell me family happiness is their highest value. However, the same person may be working a 12-hour day and getting home when the kids are in bed. This is not to say that this person's values do not include family happiness, it is just that perhaps financial security, or even achievement may be stronger for them. So, look at your actions for a true indication of your values – not what you think they ought to be.

> Revisit the list and change the order of your values if you feel it is necessary. What you should come out with is a list of your top three values. These are the things that are driving you. We will use these later when we get to goal setting.

2 Determine your beliefs

Beliefs are also statements of who you are. If your values provide the compass for your life decisions, then your beliefs form the mould into which the energy of life flows, providing the shape of your experiences. Beliefs and feelings produce reality. They are the only things that limit our experiences.

As with our values, our beliefs are formed through a process of social and personal conditioning that begins at birth. However, although they are established by external influences, they are retained by choice. We need to understand what our current belief systems are and decide whether they still reflect the life that we want to design. Also, as with values, there can be a disjunction between our true state of being and what we would have the world perceive in our outward expressions.

If you are acting as if something is the case when your innermost thoughts suggest otherwise, then it is this inner state of being that will produce your experiences. We cannot help expressing our beliefs and our inner thought processes through our outward words and actions. To find out your beliefs, look at the pattern of your life experiences.

Do the following exercise. Take a few minutes to identify your current beliefs. You may have hundreds about many different things. List them all and see which are the ones that mould your current life experiences. They fall into two broad categories and I have given a few examples of each.

Your empowering beliefs

- I like myself
- I am good enough
- My future is full of interesting possibilities
- People are basically good
- I always find a way
- I'm always lucky
- There is enough

Your disempowering beliefs

- I don't like the person I am, or have become
- I fail at the things I try
- I am not clever enough
- Life is meant to be difficult
- People are basically only out for themselves
- You get rich by exploiting others
- I'm not a person who can take risks
- I'm not worthy

The creative process is energised when there is consistency between our thoughts, our words and our actions. If you do what you say, say what you think, and think from your true state of being, you will access the energy that created the universe. But this process cannot deliver anything more than you believe yourself to be. We cannot turn out to be anything but the person we see ourselves capable of being. If we expand our thinking, our life experiences will automatically follow. Believe with every cell of your body that you can have the best, and that is what you will get.

Many people confuse their current beliefs with the truth. Your beliefs are true for you, but others will hold different beliefs about the same things and, as a result, will have vastly different experiences. Consider, for example, your belief about money. Is your belief about your ability to earn money the same as the belief of the world's super-rich? What comes first for the super-rich, the belief or the money? Your experiences are different from theirs because of your beliefs. By developing the same beliefs about money, your experiences will eventually follow.

3 Determine your expectations

The third principle of being is that of expectation. Expectation is the expression of your beliefs and values. Your expectation is the advance signal for your life events. If you expect to be happy, successful or wealthy, with confidence, then that is what you'll get. If your mental energy goes into worrying about how you will fail, then failure is what you've ordered for yourself. Whatever you expect with confidence is what you get.

This is all very well of course, but what if we have difficulty believing that we deserve the best? It is important that we ask which part of ourselves is doing the choosing in life, or setting our expectations about the things we can achieve. Those thoughts that we have about achieving magnificent, wonderful things may well be our true state of being knocking on the door of our consciousness, telling us what is possible. We often dismiss these thoughts as unachievable fantasy, but we may be ignoring the call to realise our true destiny.

This approach can make us feel guilty about desiring certain things in our lives. Yet whatever these are – happiness, a relationship, material wealth – it is possible to make them a reality. If our belief is that we do not deserve the best, this is a sure sign that our thinking is coming from the more superficial, limiting levels of our consciousness, our programmed values and beliefs. It is our mind that limits the conscious experience of the soul, not the other way around. Discipline yourself to expect positive, successful outcomes from everything you do and your experiences will eventually follow.

4 Attract what you desire

The reason that this approach works is simple: by applying it, we are tapping into the energetic nature of the universe. The principle of attraction states that energy attracts like energy. So, what you give out comes back to you – with interest! Have you ever noticed that people with money seem to attract money? And angry people tend to attract conflict and anger in others. This is the law of attraction. What you are *being*, is the energy that you send out to the universe. So if you want more of something you attract it by giving it away. By being giving we are more open to getting. This does not mean we need copious amounts of wealth to develop a giving attitude. It is the *attitude* that is more important. By concentrating on what we can contribute we will receive the flow of the same energy, and more, in return. Give what you have in abundance – your love, humour, compassion, understanding and creativity.

The rich always get richer not only because they have wealth, but also because they have developed a wealthy consciousness. Movement and change are the nature of the universe and we should consider ourselves as a channel allowing an unlimited flow of energy through our state of being. The more we block, by hoarding for ourselves, the less free-flowing it will be, and the less we'll get back for ourselves.

Understand that every belief and thought that you energise with emotion will send out an attractive charge like a magnet and will draw like energy to your life.

Apply this principle of attraction in all thoughts and visualisations. I had a friend who was looking to move into a more suitable job. The things that she visualised were to do with the aspects of a job that would suit her needs. But she also concentrated on how her natural skills and experiences would be utilised to make a valued, significant contribution in her new role. She sought a balance where she would be gaining through the process of giving. Within two weeks she had a new job offer that was more suited to her abilities and needs.

Principles 5, 6 and 7: Control your conscious thoughts

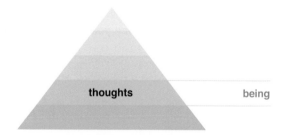

So far, we have been considering the base of the thinking triangle, that of our beliefs and values. These give rise to the next layer, that of thought, and it is with thought that the final three principles are concerned.

Thought is the starting point of all creative processes in life. Everything we see around us started life as a thought of some description. The task of painting a picture, building a bridge or writing a book, starts with the thought of doing it before any action occurs. Creating things such as paintings and bridges is an obvious example because there is a conscious intent involved.

Can our thoughts about being happy actually bring happiness? Can those about being prosperous bring wealth? The things that occur at the obvious, material level also happen at a more subtle level. We may not realise it, but those things that we think about unconsciously also eventually become form in our lives. On one level or another, we create the experiences we have through those things we think about most.

You need to direct your thought processes in a way that you are completely in charge of. However, before you can change anything you must first be aware of the thing you wish to change.

5 Increase your awareness

The fifth principle of being is that of awareness. If we are to harness and control our thought processes, the first thing we must do is to be aware of them. Earlier we did an awareness exercise based around getting in touch with our senses. You now need to apply some similar principles to your thinking processes and get in touch with how you are using your mind.

Suggesting you need to learn to use your senses may be met with the same shock that I once felt when I received a request to relearn how to drive. I was asked to attend a defensive-driving course that would supposedly make me a more aware, and therefore safer driver. I went along with an air of deep scepticism – I'd been driving for many years and already considered myself a skilful driver. This turned out to be a pitifully humbling experience as my limitations soon became evident. My tutor pointed out a completely new world, which to my surprise was significantly outside the few short metres in front of my vehicle. His anticipatory skills were breathtaking, allowing for changes in driving conditions by observing power lines and streetlights miles ahead of us. He had honed his powers of observation into an intuitive skill allowing him to recognise apparently obvious, but frequently overlooked information and to make surprisingly powerful use of it. This was a lesson I have never forgotten.

Such application takes constant awareness. Without this focused attention, our tendency is to fall into the activity of unconscious habit and the connection with conscious intent is lost. The following exercise is designed to get you in touch with your thinking processes. It is also designed to get you to make some strong associations between your negative thoughts and pain, which you can use to discourage negativity.

The elastic band exercise

Find an elastic band large enough to fit comfortably around your wrist. Each time you find yourself having a negative thought about anything - yourself, the weather, people around you - then twang the band. Two things will happen. You will force yourself to be much more aware of your thought processes, and to determine which are positive and which negative. You will also be making a direct association between negative thinking and pain. Undertake the exercise for at least two weeks and then review the results.

6 Displace one thought with another

Once aware of our thoughts we are in a position to choose to change them. The principle of displacement says that if we have a thought that is inconsistent with our desired state of being then we can substitute it for another. If a thought enters your head, and is inconsistent with what you wish to be, then *acknowledge it and do not fight it*. Allow it to pass unhindered from your consciousness. Don't give it a second thought! Then substitute that negative thought for one of your own choosing. This will take some effort at first, not to mention constant awareness. But after a while it will become second nature to monitor your thoughts and replace them with ones consistent with your vision of the future.

Exercise

Write out three positive things that you wish to achieve in the next day. For the next 24 hours think of nothing else but things that will lead you to achieving those goals. During this period, practise the law of displacement. As soon as a thought that is inconsistent with your goal occurs, let it have its moment and then follow it with a positive replacing thought. Success at this will give you an idea about how far you need to go to control your thought processes.

7 Focus on your desires

The principle of focus is this: whatever you focus on will change. Your reality is created by the things that you recurrently think about, not those that you think about every now and then. The capacity of a mind is almost limitless. If we use our mental powers like a laser beam, to focus on one thing totally and exclusively, then we can make huge changes. Because we have many things demanding our attention, we very rarely focus our thoughts on one thing at a time. Often we are worrying about the next thing. This dilutes the power of our thinking and means that we're spending our life in a future that has not yet arrived. Also, we focus on the things we don't want, rather than those we do. Get very clear about the things you do want to achieve. Whenever you feel yourself focusing on the things you are unhappy about, use the principle of displacement to substitute it for a positive desire.

Often, it is only when we experience an emergency that we put everything else aside and turn our total attention to one area of our lives. When we do concentrate with this level of intensity and intent we make huge progress. If we live and think skilfully, we apply this natural ability without waiting for the emergency.

The eleven principles of doing

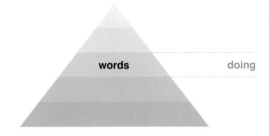

1 Use words skilfully

How often do we say what we think? How often do we do what we say? Words are the bridge between our thoughts and our actions. However, very often they are inconsistent with both of these things and as such they will dissipate our personal energy and confuse our subconscious about our desires. The key to positive creation is to have consistency between all levels in the thinking triangle. Saying what you think and doing what you say will lead to a life of great clarity.

As with your thoughts, awareness of the words that you use is a key skill. Although you may not know it, you have mental and verbal wallpaper that's a constant feature of your daily life. Find out what yours is. Listen to your self-speak and self-think, those words and thoughts that are circulating in your mind at a subtle but repetitious level.

Our thoughts occur at a subtle level that is often difficult to detect, but a clue to your thinking processes is gained by listening to the vocabulary that you use. Are you self-deprecating or critical in your words and expressions? Are you supportive or unsupportive? Do you have a positive set of words that you use habitually, or are you constantly negative?

Root out the negative words you are using and, as with the principle of displacement previously applied to your thinking, substitute them for words that are more consistent with who you wish to be. Every word that you use is an announcement of what you are, an act of self-definition. Who do you choose to be? Make the process conscious and directed.

Our words are an expression of our beliefs and values, but they are also tools for influencing these beliefs. We should therefore be careful about implanting the correct images. For example, using the expression 'I am no longer feeling depressed' makes use of the word depressed. This leaves open the possibility of retaining the negative feeling produced by this word. It would be much better to say 'I am feeling light, happy and relaxed.' These words conjure positive feelings without the possibility of misinterpretation by your subconscious.

Being positive in our words gives us positive thoughts. This is not about uttering every passing thought you have. This is about clearly articulating your truest desires and feelings to the outside world and anybody you are in a relationship with. This is about communication and delivering your personal truth without harming yourself or those around you, but at the same time utilising this creative process in a way that provides you with the things you want in your life materially and in your relationships.

Changing the words you use will eventually have an effect on the way that you think. It will change your opinions about yourself and about the world around you. Refuse to express yourself negatively. Always use positive vocabulary in your self-expression. Extend your elastic band exercise to include your words as well as your thoughts and this will help to bring your language to conscious awareness.

2 Learn through repetition

We learn everything through a process of repetition, be it a foreign language or a musical instrument. You start out clumsy and self-conscious, but once the rhythms of learning and practice are established the material quickly becomes instinctive, a part of your subconscious.

When beginning to learn how to drive, there seem at first to be a bewildering number of things to think about simultaneously. After a few months, however, things like gear changing have become instinctive, allowing the driver's conscious mind to concentrate on more important issues such as observing the road ahead. Through a process of supported repetition, a skill that originally seemed impossibly difficult becomes second nature. We learn everything through the same basic process – even our values and beliefs!

To permanently change your attitudes, we can start by managing the things that are observable. Refuse to allow anything to pass unchallenged that doesn't contribute positively to the creation of your ideal life. By consistently addressing the individual details of your mind's daily behaviour, you will quickly internalise these small changes. This will then provide a solid basis for major improvement. Through the conscious repetition of new thoughts, words and actions, you will eventually alter your values and beliefs about yoursealf and the world.

Under the principles of having, I will describe the daily use of affirmations that use the principle of repetition to alter your most deeply held beliefs.

3 Control your influences

One way to alter your thinking is to control the external factors that influence you. These include the people you choose to interact with, the things you read, the television that you watch and your general environment. Actively choose your influences and design the things that have an effect on your thinking.

For a period of one month, completely flood your consciousness with things that are consistent with the new mental attitude you wish to develop, that state of being you defined earlier. Don't buy your normal newspaper - read an inspirational book. Switch off the radio in the car and buy some personal development tapes instead. Rather than flopping in front of the television in the evening, do something completely different, or at least watch an inspirational video of your own choosing. Make a conscious decision for this period to limit the amount of time that you spend with people who do not support your own personal goals and actively seek out like-minded people with whom to build on your own ideas. After one month, notice the difference in your words and thinking and decide if you would like to make any of these changes permanent!

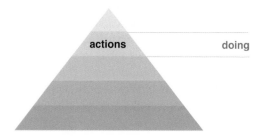

4 Take action

Everything that we have discussed up to now will have been an interesting but useless exercise unless you take action! If you are to start the circulation of creative energy in your life then you must first prime the pump. Taking action most effectively activates this flow of energy.

Activity is the expression of your being. We said earlier that everything that you do is an act of self-definition, that in every moment you're expressing who you are. Ask yourself, is this who I want to be? If not, then you can choose again, through your actions. The following principles will help you to take decisive action in your life.

5 Make real decisions

We live in a society where we are protected for the most part from significant risk and danger, where many of the accepted ways of behaving are written into a bunch of rules called laws. Where they are not explicitly stated, we have a powerful force called culture that dictates many of the unspoken rules for thinking and acting. In the minority of moments when we act of our own conscious volition, our decisions are often influenced by conditioned responses.

This means that people and organisations with an influence on culture – be they advertisers or governments – and whose interests are other than our own, can be driving our choices. We are bombarded by advertising from commercial organisations to make us think about their products in certain ways designed to lead to the act of buying. So, we are manipulated into thinking that we are making decisions about things when really we are only stating preferences between a narrow set of choices presented to us.

When was the last time that you made your own decision about something? Because the real decision making has so often been done for us, we have weak decision making muscles. The word decision comes from the Latin root *caedere*, meaning 'to cut'. A true decision cuts off all other courses of action. Once we decide to do something, we simply do it. So practise making practical decisions in your life.

6   Commit yourself to action

If you are making effective decisions then commitment will follow. When Alexander the Great set off on his campaign into Asia with nearly 40,000 men, he had enough food and money to sustain the expedition for only one month. He committed to a course of action in advance of knowing the outcome, but was willing to do whatever it took to achieve his vision. This is commitment.

One of the things that set great leaders and successful people apart from others is that they do not focus on the obstacles to achievement, but commit totally to the goal. All obstacles, whatever they are, become surmountable. Alexander knew from the outset that he'd be able to take advantage of events outside his current field of vision. This level of trust is what commitment is all about. You must be able to focus entirely on the outcome of your desires and trust in yourself so that any obstacle can be overcome.

Commitment is not just about confidence and belief, it is about action and about being willing to pay, in advance, whatever the cost of achieving your goal. You must choose with your actions as well as your thoughts. Taking action is also a powerful and clear signal to the outside world that you are serious about your intentions. Take action. Be bold and be decisive. Even if the action is not one hundred per cent right, you will be learning about the power of taking actions and seeing how amazing things will flow from that single step.

7   Take personal responsibility

Since your life is a result of the relationships in the triangle, your experiences are your responsibility. You must feel a complete sense of responsibility for every aspect of your life. Take all the credit for the things that go well and all the blame for those that don't. Regardless of the events that have occurred in your past, regardless of how you were brought up, you have to somehow leave those things behind and become the director of your own life.

Basically we can have one of two things in life: either the things that we want, or excuses as to why we did not achieve them. Many people in our culture are very adept at the latter. We have some extremely good reasons why we haven't quite achieved the dreams that we hold: my parents never supported me; I'm not in the right relationship; I've got too many people relying on me to be so selfish as to fulfil my own desires. These must be released if we are to make progress.

> Here's an exercise to see if you are making excuses. Identify a person that has overcome the same obstacles that you are encountering, and has gone on to achieve his or her dreams. They may be living or dead, known to you personally or not, but if they could do it then so can you!

8   Be persistent

This is the secret to success: never, ever give up. It's as simple and as difficult as that. Regardless of the obstacles you meet and the opinions of others, you must have an unshakeable faith in your ultimate success. This is not to say that you don't learn from the events in your life that do not produce the outcome you expected or desired. You should be flexible enough to change your approach and be forever open to opportunities to improve your creative skills. However, once you've determined the state of being that you wish to achieve, stick with it regardless of your environment. If you want to reach a state of peace, attempt to be peaceful even when the kids are screaming and the television is blaring.

Whatever your external circumstances, continue to be creative rather than reactive. If you feel intuitively that it is right and achievable for you, it is consistent with your inner most values and beliefs, then never, ever give up until it is manifest in your life. By continually facing the world from this state of being, your behaviour and even environment will eventually change too.

9   Fake it to make it

If you change the way you behave, your thoughts and eventually your belief systems will follow. As the psychologist William James said, 'thought follows action'. By altering your doing, your being will also follow. Train yourself to start behaving consistently with the vision of the new you and eventually your beliefs will reflect this new persona. See this not as pretending to be something you are not, but an assertion of your true being that has not yet found expression. So, act as if what you want is already the case. If you want to be confident, act as a confident person would. If you want to be peaceful, act as if you already are.

Faking it is not manipulation but a smoothing out of inconsistency between the levels of the triangle. It is about managing the flow of energy in your life. Whether you want money, love or business success doesn't matter – you must make a start, in any area, that will encourage the flow of energy. Rather than allow stagnation, you must consciously create a flow of energy. By acting and steadily sending energy out from yourself, you will encourage more energy to flow back in.

Of course, forcing such a change in life will at first feel decidedly uncomfortable. All change at first feels uncomfortable. If you are to reach your optimum level of performance you must get used to feeling this discomfort because it accompanies growth. Your greatest barrier to successful achievement of your personal goals is your comfort zone. We are often inclined to continue a pattern of behaviour because our subconscious is programmed to repeat the things already implanted there.

When we allow our subconscious to dictate our actions we are destined to behave as we always have done. When we do things that are inconsistent with our subconscious programming, we feel discomfort. However, this feeling of discomfort is personal growth. Get used to the feeling of discomfort associated with personal risk-taking and change.

Make a commitment to stretch your consciousness at least once each day. In Skilful Activity, I described the action of splashing your face with cold water each morning. See this as a trigger exercise to remind you to get uncomfortable during the day.

> If you seek to be supremely confident, ask yourself this: how would a supremely confident person behave in this situation? Adjust your behaviour gradually to fit this. This process is often helped by finding a role model who expresses such behaviour already.

10 Find a role model

You will not have to look hard to find somebody who has achieved the things that you desire, or who has qualities that you wish to develop. Having a role model is a powerful way of crystallising your own desires. This is not about trying to be another person; it is about developing the same level of consciousness that has brought about results in their life. If you model your approach on that of your role model, you will get the same results in your own life.

If you feel there are barriers preventing the achievement of your results, ask yourself if there is anyone who has overcome similar obstacles. If so, then you can do the same. We often block ourselves by focusing on the reasons why we cannot make progress rather than on our objectives. If one person can do something, then all of us have the same potential.

If you do not have one, find yourself a role model. It does not have to be somebody in the public eye. It may be a parent, a teacher or a friend. Make a list of potential candidates right now.

List the qualities or attributes that you admire in these people and then express them as qualities that relate to you. When you have done this, write out a personal mission statement under the headings below:

I choose to be someone who is:

These are the qualities I admire and express most:

Use your answers as your personal mission statement.

11 Clear out the old

This is a physical and mental process that will make room for the new things you wish to bring into your life.

Physical

Clear out your attic, wardrobe, desk and whatever else has been cluttering up your life for years. This may sound like a simple exercise, but I guarantee you'll feel differently about yourself and your environment once it is complete. Our outside world is a reflection of our inner workings. In this action section we are trying to use our external activities to directly affect our thinking processes. By making a change that is observable to you and to others, you are sending a powerful message to your subconscious that things are about to change.

Mental

For you to move onto the next phase of your life, it is necessary for you to leave behind everything that has been holding you back up to this point. This includes forgiving everyone and everything that you feel has caused you pain or discomfort in your life, including yourself.

The nine principles of having

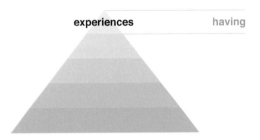

experiences   having

What do you want to *have* in your life? Better health perhaps, or more success, money and greater self-esteem? This section is about determining precisely what you wish to experience. If you don't have a clear vision at the top of the triangle, you won't be able to create – even if you're clear about the lower levels. The first few principles will be about assessing your level of motivation to change your circumstances; the rest are about being clear about what you want to achieve.

1 Assess your desire to change

How much do you want to change? Under the principles of doing we talked about commitment and decision making. The strength of these principles depends upon your level of desire. Many people do not follow through with change because their desire is not strong enough. Your desire for improvement must take you to the point of action and beyond, to a place where you will manage and overcome challenges.

However, this motivation to change must be coupled with an awareness of what must be done. Together, desire and understanding will overcome your resistance to change. This is expressed by the following simple formula:

| The desire for change | + | Understanding of the first steps | > | Resistance to change |

We are now going to quickly assess your desire, and also determine how attached you are to your current circumstances. Understanding the first steps to change will be covered in detail when we do some goal setting later.

Assess your desire to change

Take a sheet of blank paper and answer the following questions without thinking for too long. Keep them brief and don't worry if you repeat any answers.

1 What are the three key things you would like to achieve right now?

2 What would your life look and feel like if you achieved them?

3 What would you have to do and be to make them a reality?

4 On a scale of 1–10 how committed are you to taking action to change your life?

5 If it is less than 10, what are the things preventing you from taking action?

6 What are five key resources that you possess?

7 How would you behave if you were told you had 6 months to live?

8 What action could you take in the next week that would help achieve a goal?

As well as understanding your level of motivation, you also need to be clear about the things that are stopping you from moving on. On one level we get something we feel to be beneficial from our current circumstances, even if we say that we are unhappy with where we are. For example, people suffering with illness often perpetuate poor health through their thoughts because it gains them the attention and sympathy they otherwise don't get. We all get something from our current circumstances or we would not keep choosing to stay where we are.

Complete this next questionnaire to help decide if there is anything that you are getting from your current situation, even if consciously you are denying it. Often, those that strongly defend reasons for their being unable to change do so from an attachment to their current way of life.

Assess your resistance to change

Take another blank sheet of paper and again complete this exercise without thinking too hard. As before, you know the answers at some level, so keep them brief and don't worry about repetition.

1 What 3 things are you tolerating right now?

2 What do you gain from these things?

3 What have these things cost you in your life?

4 What are the things you gain from not changing?

5 What would you have to do to make decisive change?

6 What would it cost you to make these changes?

7 On a scale of 1–10 how committed are you to taking these steps?

8 Is there anything in your life you are not taking responsibility for?

Which is the stronger force, the desire to take responsible control of your life or despair at the difficulties of change? Did you find that what you are gaining from your current choices outweighs the cost of change? How you live your life is a choice. Doing nothing is also a choice, and must be made with awareness and responsibility.

2 Understand your reasons

All of our behaviour is motivated by the pursuance of pleasure and the avoidance of pain. In each moment, therefore, we are making decisions that take us away from what we perceive as being painful situations or feelings, towards those that will provide us with pleasure. However, our definition of these things is based upon our perceptions and will depend upon whether we take a short- or a long-term view. We all eat certain things that give us immediate pleasure, knowing that this is a habit detrimental to our long-term health. We may avoid addressing a destructive relationship because this will cause a fight, only to endure the pain of continuing dysfunction. Our actions depend upon whether we take a short- or a long-term view of what is pleasurable and painful.

If you are to strengthen your desire to change and to achieve your ultimate goals, you will need to be clear about the things that motivate you. You will have to have unshakeably strong reasons to achieve your goals. In one sense it doesn't matter if those forces are pulling or pushing forces, but we need to understand the difference between the two to decide if they will sustain us for the complete journey.

Pushing forces are those negative motivations that help us to avoid painful circumstances. The pain of debt, ill health and poor relationships are pushing forces that can be powerful motivators for making drastic changes. One potential problem is that such forces are reactive rather than creative. Skilful living means taking active control, without waiting for traumatic, external circumstances to spur you into action. Another challenge with pushing forces is that as the pain diminishes, then often so does the motivation for change. For example, overcoming your low energy levels by eating more healthily. Once you begin to feel vibrant and in control, it's all too easy to drop your guard and to revert to your previous habits. The best way to sustain new behaviour is to reinforce it with powerful associations with how we would like to be.

This is where pulling forces are crucial. A state of daily motivation to change can be achieved by creating a vision of the future so compelling and attractive that it pulls us out of inaction. Pulling forces are those that take you towards achievement of a goal, rather than pushing you away from a thing you wish to escape. As you get closer to that goal, your motivation increases as attainment comes into sight.

Decide right now whether you are motivated by pulling or by pushing forces. What are your specific reasons for change? To avoid staying as you are, you need to have some clear, immediate reasons for change.

Take a blank sheet of paper and complete the following:

My reasons for wanting change in my life are...

3 Be clear about your desires

Let's have a look at the top of the triangle. This is your aim: to actively create the experiences that you wish to have in your life.

Many people say to me 'I know what I want to achieve so why should I write out what I already know?' Often these are the people who don't manage to achieve their desires and live in a state of frustration, wondering why things aren't improving.

Writing out your goals displays a level of commitment and clarity that most people never achieve. Of course, if you already know your goals then the process will be easier, but the planning and preparation involved in writing them out is still crucial. It makes them concrete and real, and the process of writing will force you to think creatively. However, most people aren't clear about the things they want to achieve, only about what they don't want. In this case, goal setting is helpful because having a vague aim is the same as having no aim at all. And this is the quickest way to achieving nothing at all.

Whatever experiences you wish to have, there is nothing wrong with desiring them. This creative process is neutral and will deliver in the form of life experiences those things that are consistent with your most fundamental thoughts and state of being. As long as you understand the process of creation, you will find the combination code to unlocking your life potential. So, there is nothing wrong with desiring more money, love, success or health in your life, you simply need to go about acquiring it in a way consistent with these creative principles.

There is nothing wrong with wanting more abundance in your life, but abundance is not just about things; it is also about love, health, joy, compassion, and many of the other aspects of human existence we feel lacking. This thought that we lack anything in our lives is perhaps a reflection of an attitude that is prevalent in our culture. It may not have been expressly articulated in this way but we are taught that there is not enough of anything, so you had better get your hands on some and keep hold of it before someone else does get it! This is partly to do with our survival consciousness. Our senses are set up to be self-preserving; protecting us from attack by external sources. As a species we have survived very well up to this point relying on this instinctive mechanism. But we now live in a world where we control our environment to the extent that we have minimised many of the major risks to our existence. Our survival is better assured through cooperation rather than competition. This impulse to build barriers, to isolate or look solely after the self is actually counter productive in a world where we are totally interdependent. There is enough for everyone, so we need to develop a prosperity consciousness rather than a scarcity consciousness.

So, when you think about creating a vision for your future, don't let your cultural and biological conditioning limit your desires. Living skilfully is not a licence for self-interest to rule – once aligned directly with our true state of being, we do not need to acquire anything at the expense of others.

This next exercise is a crucial part of the life creation process we are undertaking. I want you to create a vision of how your future will look in three years' time, using the headings below as guidelines. This may be the first time you have ever done anything like this, so be expansive and ambitious.

Create a Vision of the Future

On an empty, unlined page write out the headings below. Under each write as much or as little as you like. Don't ponder for hours; be guided by your inner voice. Write things meaningful to you rather than other people's expectations of you. Remember, our thoughts dictate our experiences, so don't be afraid to push the boat out a little here. Focus on the detail of the experience as much as possible. Don't get caught up by how it will be achieved.

Paid work

This is about your ideal contribution to the world. As you write, think about:

● How consistent work will be with your personal values, passions and abilities

● Whether or not you'll satisfy your sense of achievement, pride, recognition and respect

● Whether it will satisfy your creative needs, or your physical and intellectual desires

● Your need for variety, flexibility and independence

● How well will you be remunerated

● How you'll impact upon others and the environment when you have achieved your goal.

Finances

This is about having enough resources to support the lifestyle you want.

● How will you utilise such resources, both for yourself and for those around you?

● Don't see money as an end in itself. It is the oil that lubricates the wheels of your life experiences. Have a clear picture of your cogs and wheels and the lubrication will follow. Come from a place of being, rather than a place of doing.

Material possessions

We are still trying to build an integrated picture of your ideal life, so this will include your lifestyle as well as your possessions.

● What will your day include in terms of time, activities and interaction with others?

● Where will you live and why?

● What other possessions will form part of this picture?

Relationships

This should consider all your primary relationships: with your partner, children and any others you consider important. As with all of these things, consider what you will give as well as what you will receive in these relationships. Harmony cannot exist by paying attention only to what you want.

Personal growth

Here, consider all aspects of your being - your physical, mental, emotional, and spiritual health.

● How will life be if you make these things an important consideration?

● What about education, formal or otherwise? I personally didn't see how important learning was for me until I went back to studying again.

Creativity

Is this an important element in you life? It should be, because your first masterpiece is your own life. You are creating whether you like it or not.

● How will you express yourself in life in the way that is most uniquely you?

World environment

● What things in your community, country and the world would you like to see improved?

● What would a world with these improvements look like and are there ways that you could contribute?

4 Set powerful goals

We will now discuss the part of this process that will crystallise everything that we have done up to now, and begin to make it attainable: setting the goals for your life. These are the seven distinct steps that you must follow for effective goal setting.

i Write them down

If you have not written down your vision of the future described in the previous section, go back now and write out a description of your expectations under each heading. Consider that you are painting a picture or creating a sculpture of your life in three years' time *in as much detail as you can.* Make it as complete and colourful as possible. This means that it needs to be a completely rounded, final result. Include how your typical day will look, what do you eat for breakfast, who are you waking up with, what does your day consist of. Importantly, how does it *feel?* We will talk about emotionalising later, but for now it is important that you include some *emotive* words to describe your life. You need to feel excited and passionate about its creation. This is your vision and will help your visualisations later. You now need to turn your vision into specific *goals.*

> Take a blank sheet of paper. Identify the five most important goals described in your vision. The best way to write out your goals is to describe them as if they have already been achieved. For example, 'I am doing my ideal job. It utilises my personal skills, interests and passions. My contribution is valued and I am perfectly satisfied.'
>
> These are your five key goals and describe your life in 3 years' time. You now need to break these down into sub-goals to be achieved in 2 years, 1 year, 6 months, 1 month, 1 week and tomorrow.

ii   List the benefits

What are your reasons for desiring this outcome? Get very clear about the benefits and also understand whether your motivation is powered by pulling or pushing forces. If you have a strong enough reason why, you will find a way of overcoming any challenges.

iii   Analyse your starting point

Where are you now in relation to your goal? If you are to achieve measurable benefits, you need a reference point. If you want to lose weight for example, don't focus on losing weight! Focus on your ideal weight. In other words, aim for what you want to become, not what you don't. If you want to double your sales within 12 months you have to be clear what your current performance is. Sounds simple, but many people are not clear about their starting point. Avoid comparing yourself with others in setting your targets. Top class athletes monitor progress against their personal best and success is measured in comparison to this benchmark.

iv   Set a deadline

Make this realistic but challenging. A goal without a deadline is a fantasy. Flex your deadline-setting muscles every day and you will improve your skills significantly. If you don't achieve a goal by the indicated deadline, acknowledge it, understand the reasons why and re-set the next deadline. Don't be discouraged. Use the experience as useful feedback for adjusting your approach. One of the key attitudes that set highly successful people apart from others is their attitude towards failure. First of all failure is not a word they use; results, outcomes, feedback perhaps; but not failure. There is a story about Thomas Edison being interviewed by a journalist who asked him if he had been discouraged by the 5,000 failures before he successfully deigned the light bulb filament. He replied; 'I did not fail, I simply discovered thousands of ways that wouldn't produce light.'

v   Analyse the challenges

Be clear about some of the challenges you may encounter and have a plan of action to tackle them. That way you will be less discouraged if you do encounter resistance. Once you have identified them and planned a contingency, ensure that you focus on your goal, not the challenges. Obstacles are those scary things that you see when you take your sights off the goal!

vi   Identify other resources

Firstly, it is worth listing the resources that you already have at your disposal. Your knowledge, skills, time, drive, network are all things you can utilise to help achieve your goals.

Secondly, identifying the additional resources you require may involve other people. Often the bigger your vision and goals, the more you will need to seek the support of others. This may include your family, friends, experts or your bank. The list is potentially endless. As described under role-modelling, there is great power in using the strategies employed by others. The involvement of others is often a crucial step in making an outcome more real as it can involve a 'public' declaration of your intentions. However, I would be selective, initially at least, who you share your goals with. Only disclose and discuss things with those that are supportive of your vision or are used to setting goals themselves. Most people don't set goals because they don't understand the power of the process. Stay silent about your goals to those who will not provide positive energy to what you desire

vii Make a plan

The next step is to briefly summarise all this information on the example goal-setting table on pages 114 and 115. This ensures you have all of your thinking presented succinctly in one place. Sign and date each sheet as a statement of your commitment to your new future. This is an important step and be aware of how it makes you feel.

Action Planning			
What will I do? (goal)	**How will I know it is achieved** (measure)	**By when** (date)	**Comments**

Detail Planning

Goal

Reasons why I want to achieve this goal

How will I know it is achieved

Resources at my disposal

Possible challenges	Solutions

Sub-goals and actions	Target date	Date achieved

Date by which main goal will be achieved

I am committed to following this plan and take personal responsibility for making any adjustments necessary to achieve my goal.

Signed . . . .   Date . . . .

What you should have is a set of goals and sub-goals that indicate milestones ranging from tomorrow through to 3 years' time. You now need to make this into a working plan. From now on, every activity you undertake on a daily basis should be consistent with and take you a step closer to your vision. If you keep a diary or an organiser, transfer the steps, by date into your daily activities. Before you start each day, you should know on what part of your vision you will be making progress.

5 Take action

Having a detailed plan is not enough. You must take action. Action that is entirely consistent with your goals and that persists until you get results. Your goals, vision and intentions are all meaningless unless you act on them. Action is the end of everything. Remember our change formula at the beginning of this section? This goal-setting section is simply about coming to know the first steps you will need to take, and (coupled with your motivation to follow through) should be enough to give you the impetus to overcome the resistance to change; in other words, to do something different. By doing we are working on the middle portion of the thinking triangle, but as we described earlier, we are trying to break your current cycle and alter your state of being. When these are consistent, you will be fully in control of your life experiences.

In the next week take positive, decisive action consistent with your plan. This will take you a step closer to achieving at least one of your goals. It may be making a phone call, enrolling in a class or having a conversation with somebody. Whatever it is, ensure that within the next seven days you act on something from your plan.

6 Visualise your outcomes

One of the key tools in your armoury is visualisation. Athletes, creative and business people alike develop the ability to influence results through visualisation.

When you visualise something, not only are you grooming your subconscious for success, you're also tapping into the source of all original creativity – the super-conscious. We are the active directors of the energetic stuff of the universe, and it is through our thoughts that we do this directing. Visualisation is the practice of directing our thoughts to produce the outcomes we have designed. Here are some simple rules to effective visualisation:

i Be clear about what you want

Understand that your most energised thoughts create your life experiences. Much of this section has been about aligning your beliefs with your conscious and unconscious thoughts. We often don't make the connection between our thoughts and our experiences because our thinking is ambiguous and fragmentary. By employing the principles we have described you can make visualisation work for you by bringing clarity and focus to your thought processes. Your thoughts are the mould into which the energy of life will flow to form your experiences, so be as clear as possible about the experiences you desire.

ii Change things in stages

How do you eat an elephant? The answer is *a bite at a time*! Visualisation will only work for you if your subconscious believes that what you desire is achievable.

Ophiel, a writer on creative visualisation, terms this concept the *sphere of availability*. He cites the example of a Paris rag-picker living off the city's rubbish dumps who eventually became a wealthy businessman. Initially his aim had nothing to do with starting on the road to riches. His first desire was for a small piece of carpet to keep his feet warm during cold French mornings. This *was* within his sphere of availability and was soon provided through the precise turning of the wheels of the natural creative process. Having then understood and gained confidence in the process, the beggar continued his steady ascent from there. But being firmly in the driving seat, this is a matter of choice.

The Paris rag picker *could* have set his sights on becoming a businessman with a single bound. If powerful enough, his thoughts and visualisations would have eventually provided this experience. This may have taken longer as the opportunities for such a leap would have been more limited for this man. Also whether he would have been equipped emotionally or with the appropriate skills may have been in question, resulting in an even faster loss of his acquisition than the gain.

The more gradual process offers more natural opportunities for growth to occur. Also time for the gradual acquiring of skills and adjustment of mental and emotional faculties will be available. We live in a society that values getting as much as you can as quickly as possible. Please don't misunderstand this, there is nothing wrong with rapid progress – in fact this book is about working smarter, not harder. Any shortcuts we employ however, should provide genuine, solid, lasting results, as otherwise we may find they are snakes and not ladders.

iii Visualise often

The more often you visualise the achievement of your goals, the more real they will seem. This is not about losing the power of the moment and constantly living in the future. It's about tapping into your personal power and generating a success consciousness. With this state of mind you will enjoy the present even more!

Visualisation is best done in a relaxed state. If you have ever been hypnotised, or even found yourself daydreaming, you will have been in a state of consciousness called alpha. This is a state of relaxed alertness. In the alpha state, passage to the subconscious is unrestricted and suggestions and visualisation have a powerful effect – ultimately becoming values and beliefs. This is what occurs under hypnosis. While we are in a passive state, the hypnotist can influence our thoughts and behaviour. This has the positive effect of altering certain negative and deeply embedded thoughts relating to how we see ourselves, and to certain fears and phobias.

You are the gatekeeper of your own mind. Be aware of all thoughts that pass the threshold of your conscious and allow in only those that match the image of the person you wish to be. However, more than this, the process of active visualisation sends our messages out to the super-consciousness. In other words, through this process, we are constantly communicating with the universe. Being aware of this allows us to take control of the process and to start designing the outcome, participating in the creation of the world around us.

How long and how often we spend focusing on our desires depends upon a number of variables. One single thought, if powerful and clear enough, is capable of making significant changes. However, few of us start with that kind of focus or level of desire, so doing a little every day will give the best results. Retreat to your relaxation space and spend about 10–15 minutes visualising your goals. This is not long for recreating your life! If you do have difficulty allocating a specific time during your day, do your visualisation just as you are waking or just before you go to sleep as during these times you are already in a very relaxed state.

I find that excellent results are possible using audiotape. You can easily make one of these for yourself using your own goal-orientated affirmations. Make sure you actively visualise whilst listening – don't just fall asleep! Remember, this exercise is designed to energise your thoughts, not for passive observation! Done regularly, you will find that your thought patterns start gradually to change.

Finally, remember that thinking about your goals frequently is only beneficial if they don't become a daunting obsession. So, when you do this, think of them in a light, positive way and see them as a joy, giving you greater clarity and direction.

iv Emotionalise

Visualisation is not the greatest description of the actual process as it implies the use of our vision only. All of our faculties should be employed for this process. The images that we 'visualise' should not just be pictures. We should smell, taste, touch, hear and most importantly, become emotionally involved with the object of our desire. This will make our visualisation extremely powerful.

Sometimes people have ambitious expectations of visualisation. They feel that if they do not have a full-colour TV image of a scene then they are somehow falling short. This is not the case. Visualisation works differently for everyone. But your images will improve the more you try. To see this in action, let's do a simple exercise.

Make yourself comfortable in your usual place and gently close your eyes. Use your relaxation and deepening methods (described in the earlier section on energetic light visualisation) to get you into a very relaxed state. I would like you to take me on a virtual tour of somewhere you know well, such as your home. Start at the front door and describe the front of the building to me. Point out the windows and name the rooms to which they belong. Take me into the house and then show me around each room. As we go round, explain the idiosyncrasies associated with each of the rooms - the chip on the mantel, the scuff on the wall, the crack in the windowpane. Also explain the feeling of each room - cosy, relaxed, happy, lively - its temperature, the aromas, brightness and so on. When we get to the kitchen, open the fridge and notice the lemon sitting on a shelf. Take it out and squeeze some of the juice into your mouth – feel it running down your throat, tingling your taste buds. Did your mouth start to water? Lead me back to the front door, say goodbye and then revive yourself.

Recreating a mental image of something familiar is no different to the creation of imagined circumstances. Our subconscious doesn't differentiate between reality and imagination. This means that at a deep level our emotional responses to real and imagined experiences can be the same.

To make your visualisations even more real, try and expose yourself to things that will generate at least some of the inner emotions or outer experiences of the things you desire. For example, if part of your plan is to have a new car, take one out for a test drive. You don't need to buy: you're adding a relevant experience to your sensory arsenal. If you want success, love or health, find a role model and listen to their experiences, watch their behaviour and strive for the level of consciousness they have achieved.

v Release

These are the key steps to successful visualisation. Once our clear thoughts are created, we should then release our desires to the universe and allow it to do its thing. We can get on with everyday activities confident in the knowledge that great powers are working on our behalf. We're handing over to the next logical stage of the creative process, as if asking a trusted friend to look after things.

This handing over process is not an abdication of responsibility for our life or ownership of our goals. It is simply an acknowledgement of an energetic partnership. In our visualisations we should concern ourselves only with the finished product. Visualise life when the desires have been manifest, not the ways and means of their fulfilment.

Continue your visualisations until your desire becomes manifest in your life. Once the process is mastered, results may be observed in a matter of hours or days. More complicated life changes may take longer, perhaps months or even longer, but opportunities for change and improvement will present themselves sooner. At the end of the day these are simply techniques that allow you to think clearly about, and achieve the things you wish to experience in life.

Whatever your specific results I guarantee that if you approach these exercises with sincerity and desire, your life *will* change. Your life will enhance and you will view the world around you differently. You will become more intuitive, sharper and more energetic. Your relationships will probably improve and your productivity increase as you become a more aware, alive person. You will certainly know with greater clarity what is good for you.

Through this process, these creative forces will open doors, present opportunities. It is then up to you to act upon them.

7   Verbalise

I've mentioned that repetition is a key principle in the management of your desires. Repeating your goals out loud each day is a way of soaking your subconscious in your vision of the future and assuring its realisation. At least twice a day, repeat your goals out loud and write them out, once in the morning before you are influenced by anything else and last thing at night to programme your sleeping thoughts. Keep these in a prominent place such as your mirror, refrigerator door or wallet. Look at them often, verbalise them and visualise their achievement.

> Write out your key goals as affirmations. They should be first person, present tense and as if they have already been achieved. For example:
>
> I am supremely confident, radiating a personal charisma and strength.

8   Get out of your own way!

It may be that however hard you try, you're not getting the results you want. So, let us explore some ways to improve this.

Firstly, it is important to know that the principles governing these forces are precise. For example, having a feeling of perpetual frustration about not getting what we want will produce thoughts that perpetuate this feeling of frustration. This is not a simplification, but an expression of just how exact the process is. Thinking 'I am frustrated because I never get what I want' gives you exactly that experience.

To overcome this, first decide exactly what it is you do want. Revisit the section on goal setting if necessary. You may find that this is actually somewhat confused and lacking in clarity. You may simply feel that there are a million places you'd rather be or things you'd rather be doing. But you can't have these all at once: you must choose a single desire. Be disciplined about this. As described earlier, if this is initially a small change from your current position, you're more likely to get rapid results. Once you have a good mental picture, try and let go of your frustration – it may simply be this that is causing the blockage. It won't be easy at first, but remember, energy attracts its like. Use the relaxation exercises with your visualisation and affirmations and you will find that your images grow stronger and your frustration weaker. Do this as a matter of routine. In between your exercises, think of the attainment of this goal as if it is already achieved. Don't cling on to it obsessively, seeing it as a last desperate hope of escape.

As mentioned, always give it a light, positive energy: this will ensure you don't replace one frustration with another!

Also, we sometimes have to recognise that there is a thought process within us that we've not yet changed or even identified. Declare this with a statement that may be something like this:

I acknowledge that there's something within my inner thought-processes blocking my progress towards my desire. This is not a natural part of me. I am unaware of any energy keeping it alive and causing it to manifest unwanted things in my life. I release this imperfection and feel the perfect creative forces of nature flow through me unhindered.

As you go about your daily activities, take note of how nature works without frustration, without overload. Removing this unwanted thought process is well within its capability.

Often, a barrier for us in trying to improve our thought processes is that perfect, clear thoughts seem an impossibility. It is easy for us to think that we aren't worthy to direct the sublime forces of nature. However, even though our thoughts and behaviour reflect our accumulated experience, our spirit is pure. It is true that we are seldom capable of perfection, but that should not stop us from striving towards this goal. Seeing ourselves as part of the natural, integrated universe can help to produce free-flowing visual images. If you do have difficulty with improving your thought processes, see yourself as simply a channel for the pure, perfect thoughts of the universe. We may not be capable of perfect thoughts, but nature is. Work from the premise that we have the seed of perfection within: our job is to allow it to grow. Consider the universe as trying to think its thoughts through us. It is our task to present the open frame of mind that allows this to happen. The force that causes the sun to rise every morning and the stars to come out every night will complete our tasks with the same effortless power. Make this mental analogy a regular part of your visualisations.

If we observe nature around us, we see that growth occurs gradually. There is a perfect time for everything so we shouldn't keep checking in to see how things are going. It is like uprooting a flower, just to see how well it is growing. If we are forever checking to see if a solution is knocking on the front door, we may miss it coming through the back window. Trust that this invisible force is working on your behalf.

9 Celebrate success

When you have completed a goal or a desire is realised, it is important to close the creative loop by acknowledging this. Understand your part in its creation and celebrate. Take yourself out for a meal or take a break away from your normal activities. Check the success off on your goal-setting plan. This will ensure you feel a sense of achievement and completeness.

Ensure that when a goal is achieved, you'll be ready to begin on the next. Often people lose momentum after an achievement because their approach to the next target is unplanned.

Remember, there are no mistakes. If the things you ask for are achieved and yet don't provide the fulfilment you desire, simply choose again. Keep on until you meet your true self somewhere along the path.

Thinking – Key Skills

● Know your current values and beliefs and decide whether they provide the life experiences you want

● Be specific about what you want to be: happy, prosperous, loving etc

● Carry your state of being into everything that you are doing

● Strive for alignment of all layers of the skilful triangle: thoughts – words – actions

● Be aware as to how these relationships occur in your own life

● Take responsibility for everything that occurs in your life – your thoughts will create your experiences

● Be clear about what you want to achieve – have a vision

● Set goals and frequently visualise their achievement

● Write and state your goals as affirmations every day

● Commit to taking decisive action and don't quit until you have results

● Don't be constrained by the past or by the expectations of others

● Have a vision of the future, but concentrate on your state of being right now

● Once alignment has occurred and you are in the desired state of being, surrender all expectations and trust that the process will work for you

● Celebrate your successes.

Living an integrated life

Only by integrating all the aspects of your life will you be able to meet your full potential. You were designed to live without constraint and only when this sense of freedom is achieved will you truly be living skilfully. Your health is the foundation for this way of life. You can only optimise your personal energetic resources by treating your body in the way that it was designed – by eating and acting skilfully. You will only optimise your mental, creative and spiritual resources by thinking skilfully.

Striving for mastery of these principles brings a sense of wonder and excitement, as the interconnection of everything in life becomes evident. The more one understands and experiences, the more one sees of the underlying order. Often, only through the process of looking back do we recognise that every event, thought or meeting is a piece of a jigsaw. This is where the excitement and beauty of life can be most acutely experienced. Living in the present with such understanding is one sign of mastery.

We must also recognise our integration with everything around us. Ultimately we are all connected. We are all one. Once the human race embraces this, we will take an enormous leap forward in the development of consciousness. Our current mindset is still observably geared towards individual survival. We continue to cling obsessively to our concepts of individual and national ownership. This runs counter to the needs of a world where biological survival is less of a priority than the efficient shared use of our resources. Shifting from an *every man for himself*, or *survival of the fittest* mentality to a more open, integrated consciousness will mean benefits for all.

I once heard a story from a lawyer who used to teach negotiation skills. As a serviceman at the end of World War II he was in an aircraft as an observer with a number of other officers. The pilot demonstrated the performance of the aircraft as the engines were shut down one after the other. There was some nervousness as the last engine was shut off but the pilot assured them it was possible to restart. However, the pilot had overlooked the fact that the starting motor was driven either by the other engines, or by an external generator on the ground. Consequently, he could not restart the engines. Everyone looked around at each other in terror as the situation sank in. One of the inspectors then blurted out, 'Well sonny, you do have a problem now don't you.'

Needless to say, they did get down safely to tell the tale. The pilot remembered the existence of an auxiliary generator and got the engines started again. However, many of us have the same attitude as the flight inspector. We look for someone else to blame and try to externalise the situation. But often his problem is our problem and we cannot just walk away. Such are the circumstances we find ourselves in today. The problems in the world will not be solved by nations building walls at their borders and trying to ignore the have-nots. This integration is at both individual and group levels, so we can strive for this personally by seeking for our individual purpose.

We each have a true purpose that once discovered will suddenly and totally transform our life. Find the purpose of your soul. You will know you have found it because your physical, emotional and spiritual energies will align and your life will be joyful and harmonious.

My final words to you are to wish you well on your journey of self-discovery. Remember there are no wrong turns or wasted moments. I would love to hear of your experiences along the way, as it is these endeavours that help us remember who we really are.

I leave you with a Sufi teaching story from Idries Shah's *Tales of the Dervishes*. This beautiful story is current in verbal tradition in many languages, almost always circulating among dervishes and their pupils. It was used in Sir Fairfax Cartwright's *Mystic Rose from the Garden of the King*, published in Britain in 1899. The present version is from Awad Afifi the Tunisian, who died in 1870.

The Tale of the Sands

A stream, from its source in far-off mountains, passing through every kind and description of countryside, at last reached the sands of the desert. Just as it had crossed every other barrier, the stream tried to cross this one, but it found that as fast as it ran into the sand, its waters disappeared.

It was convinced, however, that its destiny was to cross this desert, and yet there was no way. Now a hidden voice, coming from the desert itself, whispered: The wind crosses the desert, and so can the stream.

The stream objected that it was dashing itself against the sand, and only getting absorbed. The wind could fly, and this was why it could cross a desert.

'By hurtling in your own accustomed way you cannot get across. You will either disappear or become a marsh. You must allow the wind to carry you over, to your destination.'

But how could this happen? 'By allowing yourself to be absorbed in the wind.'

This idea was not acceptable to the stream. After all, it had never been absorbed before. It did not want to lose its individuality. And, once lost, how was it to know that individuality could ever be regained?

'The wind', said the sand, 'performs this function. It takes up water, carries it over the desert, and then lets it fall again. Falling as rain, the water once more becomes a river.'

'How can I know that this is true?'

'It is so, and if you do not believe it, you cannot become

more than a quagmire, and even that could take many, many years; and it certainly is not the same as a stream.'

'But can I not remain the same stream that I am today?'

'You cannot in either case remain so,' the whisper said. 'Your essential part is carried away and forms a stream again. You are called what you are even today because you do not know which part of you is the essential one.'

When he heard this, certain echoes began to arise in the thoughts of the stream. Dimly, he remembered a state in which he – or some part of him, was it? – had been held in the arms of a wind. He also remembered – or did he? – that this was the real thing, not necessarily the obvious thing, to do.

And the stream raised his vapour into the welcoming arms of the wind, which gently and easily bore it upwards and along, letting it fall softly as soon as they reached the roof of a mountain, many, many miles away. And because he had had his doubts, the stream was able to remember and record more strongly in his mind the details of the experience. He reflected, 'Yes, now I have learned my true identity.'

The stream was learning. But the sands whispered: 'We know, because we see it happen day after day: and because we, the sands, extend from the riverside all the way to the mountain.'

And that is why it is said that the way in which the stream of life is to continue on its journey is written in the sands.

Reprinted by permission from *Tales of the Dervishes* by Idries Shah (Octagon Press Ltd. London)